Essential Oils List and Benefits

MAGGIE WALLACE

First published in 2020
Imprint: Independently published

Copyright © Maggie Wallace
All rights reserved
ISBN 9798601305976

Contents

Introduction 5

Using Essential Oils Safely 7

Ambrette Seed Absolute 8
Amyris 10
Angelica Root 12
Anise 14
Anthopogon 16
Atlas Cedarwood 18
Balsam 20
Basil 22
Bay 24
Beeswax 26
Benzoin 28
Bergamot Mint 30
Black Spruce 32
Blood Orange 34
Blue Cypress 36
Bois de Rose 38
Cade 40
Cajeput 42
White Camphor 44
Cananga 46
Cannabis 48
Caraway Seed 50
Cardamom 52
Carrot Seed 54
Cassia 56
Catnip 58
Chamomile 60
Coriander Seed 62
Cinnamon 64
Cistus 66
Citronella 68
Clary Sage 70
Clove Bud 72
Coffee 74
Cornmint 76
Cubeb 78
Cumin 80
Cypress 82
Davana 84
Dill 86
Dalmatian Sage 88
Douglas Fir 90
Elemi 92
Eucalyptus Globulus 94
Fennel 96
Fragonia 98
Frankincense 100
Galbanum 102
Geranium 104
German Chamomile 106
Ginger 108
Grapefruit 110
Hinoki 112
Ho Leaf 114
Ho Wood 116
Hong Kuai 118
Hops 120
Hyssop 122
Immortelle 124
Jasmine 126
Jatamansi 128
Java Pepper 130
Juniper Berry 132
Labdanum 134

Laurel Leaf	136	Pine, Pinyon	208
Lavender	138	Pine, Scotch	210
Lemon	140	Pink Pepper	212
Lemon Balm	142	Plai	214
Lemon Eucalyptus	144	Ravensara	216
Lemongrass	146	Ravintsara	218
Lemon Myrtle	148	Rhododendron	220
Lemon Tea Tree	150	Rock Rose	222
Lime	152	Roman Charmomile	224
Linden Blossom	154	Rose	226
Mandarin	156	Rosemary	228
Manuka	158	Rosewood	230
Marjoram	160	Sage, Clary	232
May Chang	162	Sandalwood	234
Melissa	164	Saro	236
Myrrh	166	Tagetes	238
Myrrh, Sweet	168	Tangerine	240
Myrtle	170	White Camphor	242
Myrtle, Lemon	172		
Nard	174	**References**	**245**
Neroli	176		
Niaouli	178		
Oakmoss	180		
Olibanum	182		
Opoponax	184		
Orange, Blood	186		
Orange, Sweet	188		
Oregano	190		
Palmarosa	192		
Palo Santo	194		
Parsley	196		
Patchouli	198		
Pepper, Black	200		
Pepper, Pink	202		
Petitgrain	204		
Pimento Berry/Leaf	206		

Introduction

Essential oils are the highly concentrated version of the natural oils in plants. Getting essential oils from plants is done with a process called distillation, most commonly distillation by steam or water, where many parts of the plants are being used, including the plant roots, leaves, stems, flowers, or bark.

After distillation, the outcome is a highly concentrated portion of essential oil, which will have the characteristic fragrance and properties of the plant from which it was extracted, and contain the true essence of the plant it came from. This includes the smell, but also the plant's healing properties and other plant characteristics.

You can see how this highly potent extract of a plant or herb can be extremely useful for many purposes.

Essential oils have been used throughout history in many cultures for their medicinal and therapeutic benefits.

The aim of this guide is to provide a quick reference to the most common essential oils, giving its readers better access to information on the move.

Using Essential Oils Safely

Essential oils are highly concentrated substances and improper use of them can have serious consequences for your health.

Essential oils are volatile oils extracted from plants which only produce a minute quantity of oil. They aren't naturally oily plants and the volatile oils contained end up being highly concentrated. As such, most are skin irritants and harmful if applied directly on the skin, with few exceptions.

Most essential oils should **not be** consumed. They can irritate the stomach or contain unmeasured chemical compounds that are potentially dangerous.

Each essential oil has their own usage and dilution rates. This will vary from oil to oil and even brand to brand. Some oils are not suitable for skin at all or have restricted usage on skin.

Before using any Essential Oil Consult Your Doctor

If you are concerned about using a specific oil, it's important to consult your doctor. Your doctor can tell you if it's safe to use and if a specific oil is likely to affect any prescribed medications. Also take into account any allergies you have and how essential oils may affect them.

Important tips on how you can use essential oils safely:

1. Always dilute essential oils. Pure essential oils can cause serious irritation. Dilution of essential oils to 2% (2 ml of a pure essential oil to 98 ml of a vegetable oil) is considered to be optimal.

2. Do not use essential oils on sensitive areas – eyes, ears, genitals, and mucous membranes. If accidentally an essential oil got into your eye, rinse it with any vegetable oil from your kitchen. Never use water – essential oils are not soluble in water, so it will not help you. If the burning feeling or discomfort does not fade away, immediately contact a doctor.

3. Essential oils are extremely concentrated substances and excessive use of them might cause headache, nausea and other negative consequences. If you spilled an essential oil, remove it with a cloth (put on household gloves to protect your skin) and open the windows to ventilate the room.

4. Do not consume essential oils. Even though some studies highlight benefits of internal use of essential oils, the optimal dosage, possible side effects and contraindications are yet to be determined.

5. If you are a mother-to-be: be aware that some essential oils, for example, rosmarine (Rosmarinus officinalis), anise (Pimpinella anisum) must not be used at all during pregnancy because they can cause miscarriage.

6. Do not use essential oils on infants, children, pregnant women, the elderly, or those with serious health problems, without advanced medical study.

7. Use only good quality essential oils. If you use them for personal care, remember that essential oil of bad quality will not do any good to your skin and can cause a serious allergic reaction.

Ambrette Seed Absolute

Abelmoschus moschatus / Hibiscus abelmoschus

The warm, exotic aroma of Ambrette Seed Absolute Essential Oil is said to be an aphrodisiac. It is a very fragrant, but lovely, oil to use for a musky and masculine natural perfume.

This pale yellow colored, medium consistency oil is known, amongst other things, to greatly help with aches and general stiffness. It is also used to reduce stress levels and anxiety. It can also help with poor circulation and even low blood pressure.

Benefits and uses

Ambrette Seed Absolute is often used in the fabrication of natural perfumes and fragrances. It helps to reduce stress levels and anxiety.

It can also greatly help with low blood pressure or blood circulation. It can even be used for different aches or general stiffness.

Main uses

- Aches
- Stiffness
- Poor Blood Circulation
- Low Blood Pressure
- Anxiety
- Depression

Key ingredients

- Farnesyl acetate
- Farnesol
- Ambrettolide
- Decyl acetate
- Dodecyl acetate

Aromatic description

Ambrette Seed Absolute Essential Oil has woody and musky smell with exotic floral undertones.

Amyris

Amyris balsamifera

The gentle, woody aroma of Amyris Essential Oil has a very mild woody smell with vanilla undertones that is similar to Benzoin Absolute.

It sometimes replaces Sandalwood Essential Oil, even though the two aromas are not very alike. It is said to be an aphrodisiac in small dilutions and works well with other masculine smells.

Benefits and uses

Amyris essential oil often used in the fabrication of natural perfumes and fragrances. It can be used as fixative, and also helps with stress and congestion.

Main uses

- Perfumery/Fragrance
- Acts as a Fixative
- Coughs and Congestion
- Stress

Key ingredients

- Valerianol
- a-Eudesmol
- 7-epi-a-Eudesmol
- 10-epi-Gamma-Eudesmol
- Elemol

Aromatic description

Amyris essential oil is a thick, but sweet scent with vanilla undertones.

Angelica Root

Angelica archangelica

Angelica Root Essential Oil is a very versatile and appreciated oil. It can help fight various infections and reduce stress levels.

It is often used in aromatherapy to reduce stress levels and to have a general sense of well-being. The smell is very pleasant, and it is often used for fragrances.

Benefits and uses

Angelica Roots Essential Oils can be used for a wide variety of ailments.

It is used to help with nicotine addiction when you want to stop smoking, to combat stress and fatigue and to help fight infections. It helps digestion, kills microbes, reduce fever and acts like a tonic.

Main uses

- Coughs
- Sinus Infections
- Arthritis
- Gout
- Fatigue
- Psoriasis
- Stress
- Quitting Smoking and Nicotine Addiction

Key ingredients

- a-pinene
- Camphene
- B-pinene
- Sabinene
- d-3-carene
- a-Phellandrene
- Myrcene
- Limonene
- B-phellandrene
- cis-Ocimene
- Trans-ocimene
- p-Cymene
- Terpinolene
- Copaene
- Bornyl Acetate
- Terpinen-4-ol
- Cryptone
- B-bisabolene
- Humulene monoxide
- Tridecanolide
- Pentadecanolide

Aromatic description

Angelica Roots Essential Oils is a scent that has both woody and sweet tones.

Anise

Pimpinella anisum

Anise essential oil can easily be linked to black licorice. Even though the smell is quite distinctive by itself, it can also be used to elevate other scents, when mixed.

It can be used to alleviate symptoms from the flu or coughs. When used with caution, it is also be said to boost the production of breast milk, or even to stimulate menstruations.

Benefits and uses

Anise essential oil can be used for its distinctive and sweet odour of black licorice.

It can help with coughs and bronchitis, the cold or the flu. It can also help diminish flatulences during digestive issues. It is also often used in fragrances, especially to boost other odours.

Main uses

- Bronchitis
- Colds
- Coughs
- Flatulence
- Flu
- Muscle Aches
- Rheumatism

Key ingredients

- (E)-Anethole
- (+)-Limonene
- Estragole
- Anisyl alcohol

Aromatic description

Anise Essential oil has a fairly strong smell of black licorice.

Anthopogon

Rhododendron anthopogon

Anthopogon Essential oil is another name for the essential oil produced from Rhododendrons. Although not as popular as the other, this essential oil compliments many other type of essential oils.

It is particularly pleasing when used with Bergamot, Clary Sage, Lavender, Rose, Virginian Cedarwood, and any essential oils comprised in the citrus, herbaceous, floral and wood families. It is a good essential oil to use to diminish stress and anxiety.

Benefits and uses

Anthopogon Essential oil is great to relieve pains from sore muscles and inflammations. It can also be used when sick to help coughs and congestion, and generally to improve the health of the lungs.

It is also useful to deal with stress and anxiety, or general emotional and spiritual in-comfort.

Main uses

- Sore Muscles
- Coughs
- Congestion
- Lungs
- Inflammation
- Emotional Discomfort
- Anxiety
- Stress
- Heart Chakra

Key ingredients

- a-Pinene
- B-Pinene
- Limonene
- Delta-Cadinene
- (3Z)-B-Ocimene
- a-Amorphene
- a-Muurolene
- p-Cymene

Aromatic description

Anthopogon Essential oil can be perceived as a floral smell with sweet undertones.

Atlas Cedarwood

Cedrus atlantica

Atlas Cedar wood is said to be one of the first ever essential oils to be used. Egyptians used this very special oil in their embalming process. It is said to be an aphrodisiac.

It is a scent that is particularly enjoyable during the colder months, as it brings a sense of comfort. It blends very well with more masculine scents. This lovely aroma often brings a sense of calm, even though it can be used for many other uses as well.

Benefits and uses

Atlas Cedar Wood Essential oil can be used when sick to help coughs and congestion, especially in case of a bronchitis. It can help with the diminution of acne and arthritis.

It is also used to help with dermatitis and even to diminish dandruff. Atlas Cedar Wood also is great to bring a sense of calmness and to relieve stress and negative energies.

Main uses

- Acne
- Arthritis
- Bronchitis
- Coughing
- Cystitis
- Dandruff
- Dermatitis
- Stress

Key ingredients

- B-Himachalene
- a-Himachalene
- (E)-a-Atlantone
- Gamma-Himachalene
- Deodarone
- (E)-Gamma-Atlantone
- Himachalol, Isocedranol

Aromatic description

Atlas Cedar wood Essential oil is a scent that is woody, but sweet.

Balsam

Myroxylon balsamum / Myroxylon pereirae

Balsam essential oil has been used topically for many centuries in Peru. It is said to help the wounding process and issues like dry skin. However, you have to dilute it properly before using it on the skin.

Certain experts suggest to not use it topically at all, as the risks for injuries are too great. It is a very thick and fragrant oil that is mostly used to diffuse. It is also a great stress reliever.

Benefits and uses

Balsam essential oil is used to help a great number of skin problems like dry skin, and minor cuts and wounds.

It is also used to cure diseases like colds and the flu, and to alleviate stress.

Main uses

- Bronchitis
- Chapped Skin
- Colds
- Coughing
- Eczema
- Flu
- Poor Circulation
- Rashes
- Sensitive Skin
- Stress

Key ingredients

- Benzoic Acid
- Cinnamic Acid
- Benzyl Cinnamate
- Cinnamyl Cinnamate

Aromatic description

Balsam Essential Oil is a sweet oil with hints of benzoin and cinnamon.

Basil

Ocimum basilicum

Basil essential oil is known for its fresh scent that helps you focus and accomplish your tasks. It gives a lot of positive energy and helps you be productive.

It is also a great oil to help with headaches, which in turn helps you stay alert. This very strong and dominant scent can also be used in a blend, and it is great to combat colds.

Benefits and uses

Basil essential oil is great to help with colds and coughs, as it is said to be anti-bacterial and anti-viral.

Its strong aroma is also great to repel insects, and thus avoid insects bites. Basil essential oil can also be used to keep you energized and alert in order to be more productive.

Main uses

- Bronchitis
- Colds
- Coughs
- Exhaustion
- Flatulence
- Flu
- Gout
- Insect Bites
- Insect Repellent
- Muscle Aches
- Rheumatism
- Sinusitis

Key ingredients

- Linalool
- Fenchol
- Eugenol
- Methyl Chavicol
- Beta-Caryophyllene

Aromatic description

Basil Essential Oil is a very strong and dominant herbaceous smell.

Bay

Pimenta racemosa var racemosa

Bay Essential Oil, which can also be called West Indian Bay Essential Oil, as to be distinguish from Bay Laurel essential oil, as both have different properties.

Bay Essential oil helps stimulate blood circulation, and it is especially useful during the colder months. Properly diluted, it can also help with healing if used during a massage.

Benefits and uses

Bay Essential oil is a strong smell that can stimulate a better blood circulation.

It is also used in hair care, especially to help with problems of the scalp, as dandruff. During massages, it can also help with the relief of minor pains.

Main uses

- Dandruff
- Hair Care
- Neuralgia
- Oily Skin
- Poor Circulation
- Sprains
- Strains

Key ingredients

- Eugenol
- Myrcene
- Chavicol
- Linalool
- Limonene

Aromatic description

Bay Essential Oil has a rather herbaceous and spicy smell.

Beeswax

Apis mellifera

Beeswax Essential oil is special, because it is one of the rare essential oils that is animal based, as it comes from bees.

It is primarily used in perfumery and fragrance, even though it can also be stress relieving and calming as well.

Benefits and uses

Beeswax Essential Oil is more often that not using in fragrances and perfumes.

However, it can also be used to help lower stress levels.

Main uses

- Perfumery
- Fragrancing
- Diffusion

Key ingredients

- n/a

Aromatic description

Beeswax Essential Oil has a rich and very sweet smell with honey undertones.

Benzoin

Styrax benzoin / Styrax tonkinensis

Benzoin Essential Oil is a very thick and strong absolute that is rather hard to extract.

It has been used very often in the making of incense. It blend very well with other resinous or woody oils.

Benefits and uses

Benzoin Essential oil is great to help relieve pains from coughing, laryngitis or bronchitis.

It can also help with minor skin problems. However, it is mainly used to diffuse, and can help reduce stress.

Main uses

- Arthritis
- Bronchitis
- Chapped Skin
- Coughing
- Laryngitis
- Stress

Key ingredients

- Benzyl Benzoate
- Benzyl Alcohol
- (Z)-Cinnamyl (E)-Cinnamate
- Cinnamic Acid
- Ethyl Cinnamate
- Benzoic Acid

Aromatic description

Benzoin Essential Oil is a rich and strongly warm woody smell.

Bergamot Mint

Mentha citrata

Bergamot Essential Oil, also known as Lemon Mint Oil is fairly similar to lavender essential oil, and thus can be blended with this oil very well.

This oil is known for its relaxing, calming effects, whilst also rising the moral.

Benefits and uses

Bergamot Essential Oil is known for relieving respiratory distress, congestion, digestive problems, nausea, and sore muscles.

It can also be used to help with motivation and inspiration.

Main uses

- Respiratory
- Congestion
- Sore Muscles
- Digestion
- Nausea
- Motivation
- Inspiration

Key ingredients

- Linalyl Acetate
- Linalool
- B-terpineol
- 1,8-cineole
- Geranyl Acetate

Aromatic description

Bergamot Mint Essential oil is a fresh and sweet smell with floral undertones.

Black Spruce

Picea mariana

Black Spruce Essential oil is made by black spruce twigs and needles boiled and distilled. It is used to fight arthritis and relieve joint pain.

This particular oil was used by natives in North American and was said to have amazing healing properties. It is antiseptic and helpful for respiratory issues.

Benefits and uses

Black Spruce Essential Oil warms the skin when it is applied as it has anti-inflammatory properties.

It is great for joint pain and arthritis, or even overworked muscles due to exercise. It can also help with infection of the lungs and the sinuses when inhaled.

Main uses

- Respiratory Support
- Clearing Mucus And Congestion
- Calming Inflammation
- Soothing Sore Muscles
- Calming Muscle Spasms Including Coughs
- Immune Support
- Bronchial Infection
- Catarrh
- Sinus Congestion
- Arthritis
- Rheumatism
- Gout
- Over-exercised Muscles
- Joint Stiffness
- Muscular Strain
- Tendonitis
- Cellulite

Key ingredients

- Bornyl Acetate
- B-Pinene
- a-Pinene
- Camphene
- (+)-Limonene
- Camphor

Aromatic description

Black Spruce Essential oil smells very fresh woody and earthy.

Blood Orange

Citrus sinensis

Blood orange Essential oil is a bit more tantalizing, bright and tart than Sweet orange Essential oil.

It has a very citrus and bright smell and the oil is derived from cold pressing its peel. It can help with a variety of issues, from inflammation to alertness.

Benefits and uses

Blood orange Essential oil helps with inflammation whether it is internal or external.

It has antiseptic and antibacterial properties. It is also often used to treat depression and feelings of grief. Blood orange oil can help detox the system by flushing away unwanted toxins.

Main uses

- Colds
- Constipation
- Dull Skin
- Flatulence
- Flatulence
- Flu
- Gums
- Mouth
- Slow Digestion
- Stress

Key ingredients

- (+)-Limonine

Aromatic description

Blood orange essential oil has a fruity, citrus scent.

Blue Cypress

Callitris intratropica

Blue Cypress Essential Oil is well suited for emotional as well spiritual uses as it can promote a calming and soothing effect.

It has great anti-inflammatory properties if used when properly diluted. Its wonderful blue color makes it particularly special to use, alone or in a blend. It has been used for many years by the natives in Australia.

Benefits and uses

Blue Cypress Essential Oil is excellent for respiratory support, and particularly to help with asthma. It can also help clear up the skin if used when properly diluted.

It can also be used in fragrances, especially as a fixative. It also can add a beautiful hue, has it is blue.

Main uses

- Arthritis
- Asthma
- Fragrance Fixative

Key ingredients

- B-Eudesmol
- Dihydrocolumellarin
- Guaiol
- Gamma-Eudesmol
- a-Eudesmol

Aromatic description

Blue Cypress Essential Oil is woody but sweet with a fruity undertone.

Bois de Rose

Aniba rosaeodora

Bois de Rose Essential Oil is also known as Rosewood Essential Oil. It is an extremely versatile oil that blends particularly well with woody and citrus oils.

It can also be used with more spicy and herbaceous oils. It is great when used for fragrances and perfumes, as it is sweet and floral.

Benefits and uses

Bois de Rose Essential Oil can help with minor skin problems, eczema and acne. It can also relieve in-comfort from insect bites, psoriasis, scarring and stings.

It can help with tonsillitis and coughs, as well as bronchitis. This polyvalent oil also helps with stress, anxiety and depression.

Main uses

- Bronchial Infection
- Tonsillitis
- Cough
- Stress Headache
- Convalescence
- Acne
- Eczema
- Psoriasis
- Scarring
- Insect Bites
- Stings
- Nervousness
- Depression
- Anxiety
- Stress

Key ingredients

- Linalool
- a-Terpineol
- (Z)-Linalool Oxide
- (E)-Linalool Oxide
- 1,8-Cineole

Aromatic description

Bois de Rose Essential Oil is subtle but very sweet and fruity.

Cade

Juniperus oxycedrus

Cade Essential Oil is used in some cosmetic products and skin care , as well as incense. It has some antiseptic and anti-parasitic properties and can help treat dermatitis, eczema, psoriasis, scalp infections with hair loss, herpes.

Its strong musky woody aroma can promote a sense of calm and help relieve stress and worries.

Benefits and uses

Cade Essential Oil It has some antiseptic and anti-parasitic properties and can help treat dermatitis, eczema, psoriasis, scalp infections with hair loss, herpes. It can also help dandruff.

Main uses

- Cuts
- Dandruff
- Dermatitis
- Eczema
- Spots

Key ingredients

- delta-Cadinene
- Torreyol
- Epicubenol
- Zonarene
- B-Caryophyllene

Aromatic description

Cade Essential Oil has a very strong but pleasant smoky smell.

Cajeput

Melaleuca leucadendron

Cajeput Essential Oil is a particularly useful addition to your arsenal of oils to keep on hand for cold and flu season. It is a natural way to treat respiratory systems and to help recover from infections.

Benefits and uses

Cajeput Essential Oil is excellent for respiratory support, and particularly to help with asthma. It can help with tonsillitis and coughs, as well as bronchitis.

It could also provide support to diminish inflammations. It also helps with oily skin.

Main uses

- Asthma
- Bronchitis
- Coughs
- Muscle Aches
- Oily Skin
- Rheumatism
- Sinusitis
- Sore Throat
- Spots

Key ingredients

- 1,8-Cineole
- a-Terpineol
- p-Cymene
- Terpinolene
- Gamma-Terpinene
- (+)-Limonene
- Linalool
- a-Pinene

Aromatic description

Cajeput Essential Oil has a slightly fruity scent.

White Camphor

Cinnamomum camphora

White Camphor Essential Oil, even though it has camphor in its name, only has a very small percentage of camphor in its constituents. It is anti-inflammatory, very soothing to the skin, and it repels insects, thus preventing insect bites. It is also useful for bruises.

This very strong aroma is perfect to use in perfumes, aromatherapy and even massage oils.

Benefits and uses

White Camphor Essential Oil is anti-inflammatory, very soothing to the skin, and it repels insects, thus preventing insect bites. It is also useful for bruises.

It is great for respiratory support and to help coughs and colds.

Main uses

- Muscular Aches and Pains
- Rheumatism
- Cough
- Bronchitis
- Colds
- Acne
- Rashes
- Parasitic Skin Infections
- Contusions
- Bruises
- Insect Repellent

Key ingredients

- (+)-Limonene
- p-Cymene
- a-Pinene
- 1,8-Cineole
- Sabinene
- B-Pinene
- Camphene
- Camphor

Aromatic description

White Camphor Essential Oil is a fresh but woody scent

Cananga

Cananga odorata

Cananga Essential Oil is very similar to Ylang Ylang Oil, but it is significantly cheaper. Thus, it is sometime used in its place in fragrances, even if it is less floral.

It is used mostly as an ingredient in different foods and in many cosmetics. It does not have many medicinal properties.

Benefits and uses

Cananga Essential Oil repels insects and helps with insect bites. It is useful to diminish stress and anxiety.

It is great for respiratory support and to help coughs.

Main uses

- Oily Skin/Hair
- Insect Bites
- High Blood Pressure
- Anxiety
- Nervous Tension
- Stress
- Fragrancing

Key ingredients

- B-Caryophyllene
- a-Caryophyllene
- Germacrene D
- delta-Cadinene
- Linalool

Aromatic description

Cananga Essential Oil is a fresh floral but woody scent.

Cannabis

Cannabis sativa

Cannabis Essential Oil does not contain the CBD or THC cannabinoids that can be found in the plant. It is also anti-inflammatory.

Most people enjoy cannabis essential oil when it is blended with other agreeable oil. The smell can be repulsive to some people, while other might really enjoy it in a diffuser.

Benefits and uses

Cannabis Essential Oil is known to be antimicrobial, analgesic and anti-inflammatory.

It does not have the same properties as the plant, as the level of CBD to THC are almost non-existent in the essential oil.

Main uses

- Analgesic
- Anti-inflammatory

Key ingredients

- B-Myrcene
- B-Caryophyllene
- (E)-B-Ocimene
- Terpinolene
- a-Pinene
- a-Caryophyllene
- B-Pinene

Aromatic description

Cannabis Essential Oil is a herbaceous and somewhat spicy scent.

Caraway Seed

Carum carvi

Caraway Seed Essential Oil is not as used as other essential oils in aromatherapy. However, it adds a wonderfully unique aroma to any blend in fragrances or perfumes.

It is a really universal oil, has its smell is pleasant to use in blends for both men and women. It can be used as an expectorant and helps with coughs and congestion.

Benefits and uses

Caraway Seed Essential Oil can be used as an expectorant and helps with coughs and congestion.

It can also relieve symptoms from the cold or laryngitis.

Main uses

- Bronchitis
- Coughing
- Laryngitis
- Colds

Key ingredients

- (+)-Carvone
- (+)-Limonene
- B-Myrcene

Aromatic description

Caraway Seed Essential Oil is sweet, but spicy with herbaceous undertones.

Cardamom

Elettaria cardamomum

Cardamom Essential Oil is often used in different foods as a culinary addition. It can also be used as a wonderful mouth refresher instead of gums or mints.

It is particularly useful in different blends, as it helps to bring out the other scents. It is a lovely uplifting and energizing scent.

Benefits and uses

Cardamom Essential Oil can help lower spasms, help with the negative impacts of chemotherapy and reduce nausea. It is also known as antiseptic, antimicrobial and an aphrodisiac.

It can also be used as a stimulant to boost productivity and positive energy.

Main uses

- Appetite (loss of)
- Colic
- Fatigue
- Halitosis (Bad Breath)
- Stress

Key ingredients

- 1,8-Cineole
- a-Terpinyl Acetate
- Linalyl acetate
- (+)-Limonene
- Linalool

Aromatic description

Cardamom Essential Oil is spicy, woody, but also sweet.

Carrot Seed

Daucus carota

Carrot Seed Essential Oil is first and foremost used for its applications in the realm of skin care. It is particularly useful in helping damaged skin.

The very strong aroma can be toned down by mixing it with other scents, as it can be somewhat overpowering by itself for some people.

Benefits and uses

Carrot Seed Essential Oil is antiseptic, disinfectant, and an antioxidant.

It is mostly useful for damaged skins and other minor skin problems. It can also be used as a tonic substance. It also can help with digestion.

Main uses

- Eczema
- Gout
- Mature Skin
- Toxin Build-up
- Water Retention

Key ingredients

- Carotol
- a-Pinene
- Dauca-4,8-diene
- B-Caryophyllene
- (E)-Dauc-8-en-4B-ol

Aromatic description

Carrot Seed Essential Oil is very earthy and woody, somewhat spicy.

Cassia

Cinnamomum cassia

Cassia essential oil strongly resembles cinnamon in its scent. As it is cheaper, it is sometimes used as a substitute for this aroma.

Very few of us actually use cinnamon, even for cooking, as it is often replaced by Cassia.

Benefits and uses

Cassia essential oil is mostly used for fragrance and perfumes. It often replaces cinnamon in such mixes.

It could also be used for indigestion, gas, colics and even diarrhoea. It might also be useful in fighting the flu or colds.

Main uses

- Fragrancing
- Indigestion
- Gas
- Colic
- Diarrhea
- Rheumatism
- Cold/Flu

Key ingredients

- (E)-Cinnamaldehyde
- (Z)-Cinnamaldehyde
- (E)-Cinnamyl Acetate
- Benzaldehyde
- 2-Phenylethyl acetate

Aromatic description

Cassia essential oil is a spicy but sweet scent with cinnamon undertones.

Catnip

Nepeta cataria

Catnip essential oil is very often used as a mosquito and insects repellent. It is also a very pleasant scent for cats, as it attracts them.

It can help stimulate your feline friend and give them a very pleasant sensation. It is also anti-microbial and antiseptic.

Benefits and uses

Catnip essential oil is used as a mosquito and insects repellent. It is also used to help reduce all types of cramps, whether they are muscular, intestinal or respiratory.

It is also used to stimulate cats, as it is very pleasant to them.

Main uses

- Anti-Microbial
- Antiseptic
- Anti-Spasmodic
- Congestion
- Mosquito-Repellent

Key ingredients

- Nepetalactone Isomers
- Nepetalic Acid
- Dihydronepetalactone
- B-Caryophyllene
- Caryophyllene Oxide

Aromatic description

Catnip essential oil is herbaceous with an undertone of mint.

Chamomile

Anthemis nobilis

Chamomile Essential Oil can greatly help anyone who might be struggling with depression, loneliness, intense fear, anxiety or post traumatic depression.

It is particularly effective in bringing a sense of calm and to reduce stress. It can also have a sedative effect, which helps to combat insomnia and headaches.

Benefits and uses

Chamomile Essential Oil is known to be antispasmodic, antiseptic, antibiotic and antidepressant, it can be used to bring a sense of calm and to reduce levels of stress and anxiety.

It can also have a sedative effect, which helps to combat insomnia.

Main uses

- Abscesses
- Allergies
- Arthritis
- Boils
- Colic
- Cuts
- Cystitis
- Dermatitis
- Dysmenorrhea
- Earache
- Flatulence
- Hair
- Headache
- Inflamed Skin
- Insect Bites
- Insomnia
- Nausea
- Neuralgia
- PMS
- Rheumatism
- Stress
- Wounds

Key ingredients

- Isobutyl Angelate
- Butyl Angelate
- 3-Methylpentyl Angelate
- Isobutyl Butyrate
- Isoamyl Angelate

Aromatic description

Chamomile Essential Oil is sweet, but herbaceous and fresh.

Coriander Seed

Coriandrum sativum

Coriander Seed Essential Oil is a very invigorating and highly stimulating essential oil. It is particularly used to help digestion, aches, pains and arthritis.

It is rich in antioxidants and is a very powerful cleanser and detoxifier. It can also be used to flavour foods, especially Mexican dishes.

Benefits and uses

Coriander Seed Essential Oil is used to help digestion, aches, pains and arthritis. It can be a great relief from stress, and an energetic support.

It can also help you detox your bodies from unwanted toxins.

Main uses

- Aches
- Arthritis
- Colic
- Fatigue
- Grout
- Indigestion
- Nausea
- Rheumatism

Key ingredients

- Linalool
- a-Pinene
- Gamma-Terpinene
- B-Pinene
- p-Cymene

Aromatic description

Coriander Seed Essential Oil is herbaceous, fresh, and slightly citrus.

Cinnamon

Cinnamomum verum

Cinnamon Bark Essential Oil is richer in scent than ground cinnamon. It is known to be warming, stimulating and energizing.

It mixes well with many other essential oils, especially citrus and spicy ones. It is a great antioxidants.

Benefits and uses

Cinnamon Bark Essential Oil is a great antioxidants. It can promote good, healthy blood circulation and help with a healthy digestion.

It can also reduce stress levels and anxiety.

Main uses

- Sluggish Digestion
- Colds/Flu Exhaustion
- Lice
- Circulation
- Rheumatism
- Scabies
- Stress

Key ingredients

- (E)-Cinnamaldehyde
- Eugenol
- (E)-Cinnamyl Acetate
- Linalool
- B-Caryophyllene
- p-Cymene

Aromatic description

Cinnamon Bark Essential Oil is bright, woody and spicy.

Cistus

Cistus ladaniferus

Cistus Essential Oil is often used as a fixative in natural perfumery and fragrancing. It blends extremely well with a great quantity of other essential oils, and it brings out their scents.

It can help you feel more grounded and at peace. It is known for its great wound healing abilities.

Benefits and uses

Cistus Essential Oil is used in anti-aging skin care and as an anti-inflammatory for arthritis and painful joints. It is known for its remarkable wound healing abilities.

It is great to fight against infections, especially bronchitics. It helps with coughs issues.

Main uses

- Antiseptic
- Anti-microbial
- Astringent
- Emmenagogue
- Expectorant
- Sedative
- Vulnerary

Key ingredients

- a-Pinene
- Camphene
- Hexen-1-ol
- Trimethylcyclohexanone
- Bornyl Acetate

Aromatic description

Cistus Essential Oil is herbaceous, woody and with floral undertones.

Citronella

Cymbopogon nardus

Citronella Essential Oil is mostly used to repel mosquitoes and other insects. However, it can also be used as a delicious flavouring for foods and beverages, especially during the warmer months.

It is known to kill bacteria and help fight depression.

Benefits and uses

Citronella Essential Oil is antibacterial, antidepressant, antiseptic, anti-inflammatory and can be used as a deodorant. It is great for respiratory support and to help coughs and colds.

It can also be used to help with fevers and fatigue.

Main uses

- Muscular Aches
- Infectious Skin Conditions
- Fevers
- Heat Rash
- Excessive Perspiration
- Fungal Infections
- Fatigue
- Insect Bites
- Insect Deterrent

Key ingredients

- Citronellal
- Geraniol
- (-)-Citronellol
- (-)-Limonene
- (E)-Methyl Isoeugenol
- Champhene
- Citronellyl acetate

Aromatic description

Citronella Essential Oil is very fresh and slightly fruity.

Clary Sage

Salvia sclarea

Clary Sage Essential Oil is very good for combating stress, and has a unique ability to ease stress and calm frazzled nerves. is considered an aphrodisiac by some.

It can blend very well with bergamot, lime, lavender, Roman chamomile, sandalwood, cedarwood, patchouli and rose.

Benefits and uses

Clary Sage Essential Oil is widely used in a number of topical, respiratory, digestive, emotional and feminine issues. It can help with flatulence, hair loss and dandruff.

It can also help with whooping cough and asthma attacks.

Main uses

- Acne
- Skin Inflammation
- Hair Loss
- Dandruff
- Dry Or Mature Skin
- Muscular Aches
- Whooping Cough
- Asthma Attacks
- Eases Menstrual Pain
- Regulation Of Menstrual Flow
- Flatulence
- Intestinal Cramping
- Colic
- Stress
- High Blood Pressure
- Amenorrhea
- Coughing
- Dysmenorrhea
- Exhaustion
- Labor Pains
- Sore Throat

Key ingredients

- Linalyl Acetate
- Linalool
- a-Terpineol
- Germacrene D
- B-Caryophyllene

Aromatic description

Clary Sage Essential Oil is herbaceous, earthy, slightly floral.

Clove Bud

Syzygium aromaticum

Clove Bud Essential Oil is formed through a distillation process from the buds of the clove tree. It is useful for use in blends with the intention to help relieve pain.

It is also a very good antimicrobial essential oil. It's recommended to use it when experiencing dental pain. Clove Essential Oil is extremely strong and using it at undiluted for any purpose is not a good idea.

Benefits and uses

Clove Bud Essential oil is invigorating and mentally stimulating. Since that is the case, research has be done regarding cognitive and brain health that seems promising.

It offers pain relief, help with bacterial infection, fungal infection, muscle pain, rheumatism, flu and bronchitis.

Main uses

- Pain Relief
- Bacterial Infection
- Fungal Infection
- Viral Skin Infection
- Warts
- Verrucas
- Toothache
- Gum Disease
- Muscle Pain
- Rheumatism
- Flu
- Bronchitis
- Tired Limbs
- Nausea
- Flatulence
- Stomach Cramp
- Abdominal Spasm
- Parasitic
- Infection
- Scabies
- Ringworm

Key ingredients

- Eugenol
- B-Caryophyllene
- Eugenyl Acetate
- a-Caryophyllene
- Isoeugenol
- Methyleugenol

Aromatic description

Clove Bud Essential Oil has a strong, warm, spicy aroma.

Coffee

Coffea arabica

The aromatic oil is within the coffee bean and Coffee Oil is often made through cold pressing coffee beans. It is sometimes by infusing coffee beans into a vegetable oil.

Its use could possibly help suppress the craving for some coffee in some people.

Benefits and uses

Coffee Extract is mostly used for fragrances and perfumes, and can also be diffused.

Main uses

- Perfumery and Fragrance
- Diffusion

Key ingredients

- 2-furanmethanol
- Methylpyrazine
- 2,6 Dimethylpyrazine
- 5-Methylfurfural
- Furfuryl Acetate
- Caffeine (< 0.5%)

Aromatic description

Coffee CO_2 Extract has a rich, strong coffee smell.

Cornmint

Mentha arvensis

Steam Distilled Cornmint Essential Oil is made as to remove a large percentage of the menthol it naturally contains. Contrary to peppermint oil, is not commonly used within aromatherapy.

It has fragrance and soap-making applications, as it is cheaper than other types of mint.

Benefits and uses

It is often used in fragrances, and generally has the same applications as peppermint oil.

Main uses

- Asthma
- Colic
- Exhaustion
- Flu
- Digestion
- Flatulence
- Headache
- Nausea
- Scabies
- Sinusitis
- Vertigo

Key ingredients

- Menthol
- Menthone
- Isomenthone
- Limonene
- Pinene

Aromatic description

Cornmint Essential Oil is very minty, fresh and menthol-like.

Cubeb

Piper cubeba

Cubeb Essential Oil resembles black pepper essential oil. However, it's a softer essential oil that is used as a middle-base note in fragrances. It blends well with other spice essential oils.

It is a great secondary essential oil for blends meant to help uplift and energize without being overly stimulating.

Benefits and uses

Cubeb Essential Oil is a great essential oil for respiratory issues, pain relief, and digestive complaints.

It can be used to help coughs, infections, colds, the flu and flatulences. It is also great in fragrances.

Main uses

- Cystitis
- Urethritis
- Leukorrhea
- Bronchitis
- Congestion
- Coughs
- Mucus
- Sinusitis
- Throat Infections
- Flatulence
- Sluggish Digestion
- Indigestion

Key ingredients

- Sabinene
- Cubebol
- a-Copaene
- B-Cubebene
- Delta-Cadinene
- a-Cubebene
- a-Pinene
- Gamma-Humulene
- (+)-Limonene
- (-)-allo-Aromadendrene
- Gamma-Muurolene
- (Z)-Calamene
- B-Caryophyllene

Aromatic description

Cubeb Essential Oil is a warm, sweet oil that is also peppery.

Cumin

Cuminum cyminum

Cumin Essential Oil has a very rich, spicy, and even earthy scent that some really appreciate.

Some would even say they find it sensual.

Benefits and uses

Cumin Essential oil is great to get rid of toxin build-up. It also helps with poor circulation, low blood pressure, colic, stomach cramps and indigestion.

Main uses

- Toxin Buildup
- Poor Circulation
- Low Blood Pressure
- Colic
- Stomach Cramps
- Indigestion
- Gas
- Fatigue

Key ingredients

- Cuminaldehyde
- Cymene
- Phellandrene
- Myrcene
- Limonene
- Farnesene
- Caryophyllene

Aromatic description

Cumin Essential Oil has a rich, spicy, earthy aroma.

Cypress

Cupressus sempervirens

Cypress Essential Oil mixes well with a many essential oils as other woody oils, mint oils, the citrus oils, most specifically grapefruit, and it is beautifully blended in low dilution with florals.

It is great when you need help to be able to concentrate.

Benefits and uses

Cypress Essential Oil is great to help improve self-confidence, willpower, perseverance and motivation.

It helps with haemorrhoids and excessive perspiration as well as oily skin.

Main uses

- Astringent
- Excessive Perspiration
- Hemorrhoids
- Menorrhagia
- Oily Skin
- Rheumatism
- Vericose Veins

Key ingredients

- a-Pinene
- delta-3-Carene
- Cedrol
- a-Terpinyl acetate
- Terpinolene
- (+)-Limonene

Aromatic description

Cypress Essential Oil smells fresh, herbaceous and woody.

Davana

Artemisia pallens

Davana Essential Oil is most often steam distilled from leaves and flowers. It is well liked and used as a natural fragrances, as well as blended.

It is a versatile oil that blends particularly well with essential oils in the wood, spice, resin, floral and citrus groups.

Benefits and uses

Davana Essential oil can help with bacterial infection, bronchial Congestion, reduce coughs, help with colds and help cure Influenza. It also helps with indigestion and nausea.

It is a great stress reliever and helps with anxiety.

Main uses

- Bacterial Infection
- Bronchial Congestion
- Coughs
- Colds
- Influenza
- Nervous Stomach
- Indigestion
- Nausea
- Menstrual Cramps
- Menopausal Symptoms
- General Debility
- Anxiety
- Stress
- Irritability
- Tension
- Anxiety
- Wound Healing
- Antiseptic
- Coughs

Key ingredients

- (Z)-Davanone
- Nerol
- Furans
- (E)-Davanone
- Geraniol
- Isodavanone
- (Z)-Hydroxy-davanone
- Davanic Acid
- Cinnamyl Cinnamate

Aromatic description

Davana Essential Oil is rich, sweet, fruity and a little woody.

Dill

Anethum graveolens

Dill Seed Essential Oil is a very interesting and rather beneficial essential oil, especially when it is used for digestive issues.

As for its aroma, Dill Seed Oil has a little earthy, fresh, sweet, herbaceous aroma that mixes particularly well with essential oils of the citrus, spice, wood and herbaceous families.

Benefits and uses

Dill Seed Essential Oil is a very interesting and rather beneficial essential oil, especially when it is used for digestive issues.

It helps with flatulence, indigestion, bronchial Asthma and the promotion of lactation.

Main uses

- Dyspepsia
- Flatulence
- Indigestion
- Bronchial Asthma
- Dysmenorrhoea And The Promotion Of Lacation

Key ingredients

- (+)-Limonene
- (+)-Carvone
- (E)-Dihydrocarvone
- a-Phellandrene
- (Z)-Dihydrocarvone

Aromatic description

Dill Seed Essential Oil smells fresh, sweet and herbaceous.

Dalmatian Sage

Salvia officinalis

Essential oil that is steam distilled and is referred to by many other names including Common Sage essential oil.

It is a great smell that blends extremely well with other essential oils in the citrus, spice, mint, wood and herbaceous families.

Benefits and uses

Dalmatian Sage Essential oil greatly helps with different aches, especially muscle aches and joint pains.

It also helps with digestive problems and flatulences. It can help with mental fatigue.

Main uses

- Muscular Aches
- Joints
- Headaches
- Digestive Upsets
- Sore Throat
- Menstrual Cramping
- Nervousness
- Mental Fatigue
- Emotional Exhaustion
- Memory Loss
- Acne

Key ingredients

- Camphor
- a-Thujone
- Borneol
- 1,8-Cineole
- B-Thujone
- B-Caryophyllene

Aromatic description

Dalmatian Sage Essential Oil is herbaceous, fruity and fresh.

Douglas Fir

Pseudotsuga menziesii

Douglas Fir Essential Oil is rather sweet, woody and very pine-like. It certainly is a very nice conifer essential oil to be using during the holidays and the colder months.

As such, it blends well with other conifer and wood essential oils. It can also act as a great fixative among other oils.

Benefits and uses

Douglas Fir Essential Oil is great to fight diarrhoea, colds and the flu. It is also known to be uplifting in spirits.

It is used in fragrances, especially near the Holidays.

Main uses

- Diarrhoea
- Cystitis
- Colitis
- Colds/Flu
- Emotionally Uplifting

Key ingredients

- Camphene
- a-Pinene
- B-Pinene
- Bornyl acetate
- Terpinolene
- Sabinene
- Terpinen-4-ol

Aromatic description

Douglas Fir Essential Oil is woody with floral notes.

Elemi

Canarium luzonicum

Elemi Essential Oil is distilled from the resin of an Asian tree.

It is also extremely helpful in taking care of wounds and for supporting respiratory health.

Benefits and uses

Elemi essential oil is extremely helpful in taking care of wounds and for supporting respiratory health.

It can also help with respiratory issues, such as repetitive coughing. It also helps with fatigue.

Main uses

- Respiratory Tract Infections
- Chronic Coughs
- Catarrh
- Stress-Related Bronchial Conditions
- Muscular Fatigue
- Infectious Skin Conditions
- Wounds
- Cuts
- Fatigue

Key ingredients

- (+)-Limonene
- Elemol
- a-Phellandrene
- Elemicin
- p-Cymene
- a-Pinene
- 1,8-Cineole

Aromatic description

Elemi Essential Oil is fresh, citrus and a little peppery.

Eucalyptus Globulus

Eucalyptus globulus

Eucalyptus Globulus Essential Oil is the most commonly available type of eucalyptus essential oil.

It is known especially for its great benefits for respiratory infections including helping to ease congestion and pressure, colds, flu, fever and bronchitis.

Benefits and uses

Eucalyptus Globulus Essential Oil is known especially for its great benefits for respiratory infections including helping to ease congestion and pressure, colds, flu, fever and bronchitis.

Main uses

- Respiratory Infection
- Bronchitis
- Infectious Disease
- Fever
- Catarrh
- Sinusitis
- Fever
- Muscular Aches And Pains
- Rheumatism
- Arthritis
- Urinary Infection
- Cystitis
- Parasitic Infection

Key ingredients

- 1,8-Cineole
- a-Pinene
- (+)-Limonene
- Globulol
- (E)-Pinocarveol

Aromatic description

Eucalyptus Globulus Essential Oil is fresh and woody.

Fennel

Foeniculum vulgare

Sweet Fennel Essential Oil is known for its ability to greatly help with digestive and menstrual problems. It can be helpful in blends as it helps with mental stimulation, clarity and focus.

It helps suppress the appetite, and thus help to support weight loss.

Benefits and uses

Sweet Fennel Essential Oil is known for its ability to greatly help with digestive and menstrual problems.

It can be helpful in blends as it helps with mental stimulation, clarity and focus.

Main uses

- Digestive Disorders
- Dyspepsia
- Gastrointestinal Spasm
- Flatulence
- Nausea
- Constipation
- Irritable Bowel Syndrome
- Abdominal Spasm
- Menstrual Problems
- Premenstrual Syndrome
- Fertility
- Endometriosis
- Menopausal Symptoms
- Cellulite
- Fluid Retention
- Heavy Legs
- Bronchitis
- Respiratory Issues
- Parasitic Infections

Key ingredients

- (E)-Anethole
- (+)-Limonene
- Fenchone
- Estragole
- a-Pinene

Aromatic description

Sweet Fennel Essential Oil smells sweet and peppery.

Fragonia

Taxandria fragrans

All oil named Fragonia, is bought from a reliable source as it is trademarked. It is highly renowned as a respiratory oil. It is also very anti-microbial. It is also used as an anti-inflammatory oil.

This Essential Oil can help enhance the dignity of a person and its emotional state.

Benefits and uses

Fragonia Essential Oil helps with many respiratory conditions, such as coughs and bronchitis.

It also helps with sinus congestion and colds. It also helps with acne.

Main uses

- Respiratory Conditions
- Bronchitis
- Catarrh
- Sinus Congestion
- Colds
- Inflammatory Muscular Conditions
- Bacterial And Fungal Infections
- Pain
- Acne

Key ingredients

- 1,8-Cineole
- a-Pinene
- Linalol
- a-Terpineol
- Terpinen-4-ol

Aromatic description

Fragonia Essential Oil smells a little bit like Eucalyptus Essential Oil.

Frankincense

Boswellia carterii

Frankincense is a tree resin is used for its medicinal, cosmetic, aromatic and spiritual applications.

It is used, most of the time, for spiritual uses, perfumes and incense / room fragrances. Some people seem to find the scent really grounding and calming.

Benefits and uses

Frankincense Essential Oil is mostly used to mix in fragrances. It is also used in incenses, in blends or alone.

It can help get a sense of mental clarity and of general calm. It helps lower anxiety and stress levels.

Main uses

- Anxiety
- Asthma
- Bronchitis
- Extreme Coughing
- Scars
- Stress
- Stretch Marks

Key ingredients

- a-Pinene
- a-Phellandrene
- (+)-Limonene
- B-Myrcene
- B-Pinene
- B-Caryophyllene
- p-Cymene
- Terpinen-4-ol
- Verbenone
- Sabinene
- Linalool

Aromatic description

Frankincense Essential Oil smells fresh, woody and a little spicy.

Galbanum

Ferula galbaniflua

Galbanum Essential Oil is steam distilled and has been used as incense and in perfumery since ancient times.

Galbanum Essential Oil is general mostly known for its anti-inflammatory, anti-microbial properties. Some people prefer it when blended, as the scent can be strong.

Benefits and uses

Galbanum Essential Oil is general mostly known for its anti-inflammatory, anti-microbial properties.

Many people find it calming as it helps lower anxiety and stress levels.

Main uses

- Inflammatory Skin Disorders
- Acne
- Pimples
- Cuts
- Wounds
- Scars
- Bronchitis
- Coughs
- Respiratory Issues
- Inflammatory
- Muscular Aches And Pains
- Rheumatoid Arthritis
- Indigestion
- Nerve-related Conditions

Key ingredients

- B-Pinene
- Gamma-3-Carene
- a-Pinene
- Sabinene
- B-Myrecene
- (+)-Limonene

Aromatic description

Galbanum Essential Oil smells fresh, greenish and earthy.

Geranium

Pelargonium graveolens

Geranium Essential Oil is most often used for women, due to its very floral smell. It is also very useful in helping the reproductive system, menstrual cycle and the menopause. It can also be very helpful with haemorrhoids and even varicose veins.

Geranium Essential Oil blends especially well with essential oils in the citrus, floral, wood and mint families.

Benefits and uses

Geranium Essential Oil is very useful in helping the reproductive system, menstrual cycle and the menopause in women. It can also be very helpful with haemorrhoids and even varicose veins.

It also helps with depression and fatigue.

Main uses

- Female Reproductive Disorders
- Menstrual Cramps
- Endometriosis
- Premenstrual Syndrome
- Menopausal Symptoms
- Circulatory Disorders
- Reynaud's Disease
- Varicose Veins
- Haemorrhoids
- Neuralgia
- Depression
- Emotional Crisis
- Stress
- Wounds
- Acne
- Dermatitis
- Eczema
- Ulcers

Key ingredients

- Citronellol
- Geraniol
- Linalol
- Citronellyl formate
- 10-epi-Gamma-Eudesmol
- Geranyl Formate
- Isomenthone

Aromatic description

Geranium Essential Oil smells floral, fresh and sweet.

German Chamomile

Matricaria recutita

German Chamomile oil is a great anti-inflammatory oil to use in topical applications.

It has is a deep, dark blue hue.

Benefits and uses

German Chamomile Essential oil helps with many minor skins problems, as acne.

It can also be used for coughs, insomnia, flatulences, digestive issues, and many other problems.

Main uses

- Abscesses
- Allergies
- Arthritis
- Boils
- Colic
- Cystitis
- Dermatitis
- Dysmenorrhea
- Ear Ache
- Flatulence
- Hair
- Headache
- Inflamed Skin
- Insect Bites
- Insomnia
- Nausea
- Neuralgia
- PMS
- Rheumatism
- Sores
- Stress
- Wounds

Key ingredients

- Bisabolol
- Farnesol
- Azulene
- Farnasene
- Thujanol

Aromatic description

German Chamomile Essential Oil smells sweet, fruity and herbaceous.

Ginger

Zingiber officinale

Ginger Essential Oil can be great in blends which help improve blood circulation. We often see them in blends for massage.

It is energizing and uplifting in spirits. It can thus help with productivity.

Benefits and uses

Ginger Essential Oil can be great in blends which help improve blood circulation.

It is also very useful for aching muscles and arthritis. It is also great for indigestion.

Main uses

- Aching Muscles
- Arthritis
- Nausea
- Indigestion
- Poor Circulation
- Nervous Exhaustion

Key ingredients

- Zingiberene
- ar-Curcumene
- B-Sesquiphellandrene
- B-Bisabolene
- Camphene
- B-Phellandrene
- Borneol
- 1,8-Cineole
- a-Pinene
- B-Elemene

Aromatic description

Ginger Essential Oil is spicy and warming.

Grapefruit

Citrus paradisi

Grapefruit Essential Oil blends well with many other essential oils.

It is a greatly energizing oil that isn't too strong and that will not overpower everything. It helps with sweetening blends.

Benefits and uses

Grapefruit essential oil is great to help with acne, oily skin, cellulite and skin that needs a little more shine.

It also helps with water retention.

Main uses

- Acne
- Oily Skin
- Cellulitis
- Dull Skin
- Toxin Build-up
- Water Retention
- Nervous Exhaustion

Key ingredients

- (+)-Limonene
- B-Myrcene
- a-Pinene
- Sabinene
- Nootkatone
- Bergapten

Aromatic description

Grapefruit Essential Oil smells of citrus.

Hinoki

Chamaecyparis obtusa

Hinoki Essential Oil is available in limited quantities as a wood oil, root oil and needle (leaf) oil.

We have to be careful when using this oil, as Hinoki's quantity has lowered.

Benefits and uses

Hinoki Essential oil has Anti-asthmatic, Antibiotic and Anti-inflammatory properties.

It can also greatly help with anxiety and hair growth.

Main uses

- Possible Neuroprotective Affects Against AB1-40
- Anti-asthmatic
- Antibiotic
- Anti-inflammatory
- Anxiety
- Hair Growth
- Immune Stimulant
- Insecticidal

Key ingredients

- Elemol
- a-Terpinyl Acetate
- Gamma-Eudesmol
- Bornyl Acetate
- B-Eudesmol
- Gamma-Muurolene
- a-Eudesmol
- B-Cedrene
- a-Muurolene
- (+)-Limonene
- Delta-Cadinene
- B-Pinene
- a-Fenchol

Aromatic description

Hinoki Essential Oil smells woody and sweet.

Ho Leaf

Cinnamomum camphora

Ho leaf essential oil is often times known as Ravintsara Essential Oil and it is similar to Eucalyptus oil.

It is distilled from the leaves of the same plant that gives a great variety of camphor oils.

Benefits and uses

Ho leaf essential oil can help with influenza and general helps to support the immune system.

It also helps with stress, anxiety and fatigue. It also promotes sleep.

Main uses

- Influenza
- Shingles
- Supports the Immune System
- Stress
- Depression
- Calms the Nerves
- Promotes Sleep
- Muscular Aches and Pains

Key ingredients

- 1,8-Cineole
- Sabinene
- a-Terpineol
- a-Pinene
- B-pinene
- Safrole
- Methyleugenol

Aromatic description

Ho leaf essential oil smells fresh and earthy.

Ho Wood

Cinnamomum camphora var linalool

Ho Wood Essential Oil is distilled from the leaves of Cinnamomum camphora.

It is said to be a very calming oil, as it promotes positive calming energies. It resembles Rosewood oil and can sometimes be used as a substitute for this oil.

Benefits and uses

Ho wood essential oil is great to help with flu and colds and even influenza.

It also helps with the care of wounds and cuts, as well as acne and eczema. It also reduces stress and anxiety.

Main uses

- Colds/Flu
- Menstrual Cramps
- Wounds
- Cuts
- Eczema
- Acne
- Stress
- Anxiety

Key ingredients

- Linalol

Aromatic description

Ho wood essential oil smells fresh, sweet and fruity.

Hong Kuai

Chamaecyparis formosensis

Taiwan Hinoki Essential Oil is steam distilled from the twigs and wood.

It mixes very well with other woody essential oils, as well as citrus and floral essential oils.

Benefits and uses

Hinoki Essential oil has Anti-asthmatic, Antibiotic and Anti-inflammatory properties.

It can also greatly help with anxiety and hair growth. It is mostly used in fragrances mixed with other oils.

Main uses

- Muscular Spasms
- Respiratory Conditions
- Cramps
- Menstrual Issues
- Headache
- Mental and Physical Fatigue

Key ingredients

- Eugenol
- 1,8-Cineole
- Estragole
- B-Bisabolene
- (Z)-a-Bisabolene

Aromatic description

Taiwan Hinoki Essential Oil has a sharp but very woody scent.

Hops

Humulus lupulus

Hop Essential Oil can be found to be a bit too bitter for some people. It is often used in beers.

It mixes especially well with most essential oils including the woods, florals, citrus, spice and herbaceous oils. It is great to use in fragrances and in natural deodorants.

Benefits and uses

Hops Essential Oil is known to be used as a sedative and can be really helpful in situations of anxiety, stress and insomnia.

It can also be used as a natural deodorant.

Main uses

- Sedative
- Anxiety
- Stress
- Nervousness
- Insomnia
- Neuralgia
- Bruising
- Menstrual Issues

Key ingredients

- a-Caryophyllene
- B-Myrcene
- B-Caryophyllene
- gamma-Cadinene
- delta-Cadinene
- a-Muurolene

Aromatic description

Hops Essential Oil smells fresh and sweet with herbaceous undertones.

Hyssop

Hyssopus officinalis var. decumbens

Hyssop Essential Oil is fresh, earthy, fruity, woody and a little sweet.

It mixes really well with essential oils in the citrus, floral, wood, herbal and medicinal families. It is said to purify and cleanse you emotionally and even spiritually.

Benefits and uses

Hyssop Essential Oil is great to help with any problem of respiratory nature and can also be greatly helpful for digestion and muscular and joint pain.

It can help with coughs and bronchitis as well as colds and influenza.

Main uses

- Coughs
- Colds
- Influenza
- Bronchitis
- Catarrh
- Asthma
- Bronchial Infections
- Contusions
- Bruising
- Wounds
- Arthritis
- Rheumatism
- Muscular Aches and Pains
- Digestive Problems

Key ingredients

- Linalol
- 1,8-Cineole
- (+)-Limonene
- Gamma-Pinene
- Caryophyllene Oxide

Aromatic description

Hyssop Essential Oil is fresh, earthy and fruity.

Immortelle

Helichrysum italicum

Immortelle Essential Oil is also known as Helichrysum oil or Everlasting essential oil. It is actually a really great anti-inflammatory.

It mixes really well with Lavender, Roman Chamomile, Clary Sage, Frankincense, Juniper Berry, Virginian Cedarwood or Sweet Orange.

Benefits and uses

It is great with helping with muscular aches and pains, burns, cuts, eczema, irritated skin, wounds and infections in general.

It is then suggested to use it topically.

Main uses

- Muscular Aches And Pains
- Abscesses
- Acne
- Boils
- Burns
- Cuts
- Dermatitis
- Eczema
- Irritated Skin
- Wounds
- Nervous Exhaustion

Key ingredients

- a-Pinene
- Gamma-Curcumene
- Neryl Acetate
- B-Selinene
- Italidione I
- B-Caryophyllene
- ar-Curcumene
- Italicene

Aromatic description

Helichrysum Essential Oil smells fresh, earthy and slightly herbaceous.

Jasmine

Jasminum grandiflorum

Jasmine Absolute has a delicious floral aroma that is really unique and special. Since it is an absolute a small quantity can go a really long way.

It is said to be an aphrodisiac and to help fight against depression.

Benefits and uses

Jasmine absolute can greatly help in fighting against depression.

It is also useful for dry skin, sensitive skin and even labour pains.

Main uses

- Depression
- Dry Skin
- Exhaustion
- Labor Pains
- Sensitive Skin

Key ingredients

- Benzyl acetate
- Benzyl benzoate
- Phytol
- Squalene 2,3-oxide
- Isophytol
- Phytyl acetate
- Linalool
- Squalene
- Geranyl linalool
- Indole
- (Z)-Jasmone
- Eugenol

Aromatic description

Jasmine Absolute is a deep, rich, floral and exotic scent.

Jatamansi

Nardostachys jatamansi

Jatamansi Essential Oil is also known as Spikenard Essential Oil. It is made by steam distilling the roots of Nardostachys jatamansi.

It mixes very well, but you have to be careful, as it can overpower some of the other scent, as it is very powerful. Spikenard Essential Oil is calming and relaxing; it is sometime used to help with sleep and relaxation.

Benefits and uses

Spikenard Essential Oil is calming and relaxing; it is sometime used to help with sleep and relaxation.

It is great for meditation, prayer and other spiritual uses. It can help with insomnia, menstrual cycle regulation and menstrual pains.

Main uses

- Insomnia
- Menstrual Problems
- Muscular Spasm
- Muscular Contractions
- Neuralgia
- Sciatica
- Bodily Congestion
- Aging Skin
- Physical Tension
- Stress-related Conditions
- Anxiety
- Nervous Tension
- Soothing
- Calming

Key ingredients

- Nardol
- Formic Acid
- a-Selinene
- Dihydro-B-ionone
- Nardol Isomer
- Selinene Isomer
- Propionic Acid
- B-Caryophyllene
- Cubebol

Aromatic description

Spikenard Essential Oil is deep, rich, earthy and woody.

Java Pepper

Piper cubeba

Java Pepper Essential Oil is also known as Cubeb Essential Oil. It is a great essential oil to try for respiratory problems, pain relief, and digestive problems.

It is great as a middle-base note in fragrances and perfumes. It is very calming and it helps balance emotional issues.

Benefits and uses

Java Pepper Essential Oil is a great essential oil for respiratory issues, pain relief, and digestive complaints.

It can be used to help coughs, infections, colds, the flu and flatulences. It is also great in fragrances.

Main uses

- Cystitis
- Urethritis
- Leukorrhea
- Bronchitis
- Congestion
- Coughs
- Mucus
- Sinusitis
- Throat Infections
- Flatulence
- Sluggish Digestion
- Indigestion

Key ingredients

- Sabinene
- Cubebol
- a-Copaene
- B-Cubebene
- Delta-Cadinene
- a-Cubebene
- a-Pinene
- Gamma-Humulene
- (+)-Limonene
- (-)-allo-Aromadendrene
- Gamma-Muurolene
- (Z)-Calamene
- B-Caryophyllene

Aromatic description

Jave Pepper Essential Oil is a warm and sweet.

Juniper Berry

Juniperus communis

Juniper berries essential oil has been used for many centuries now. It is used for medicinal issues and some people even use the berries to burn them to cleanse and purify the air in their house.

Some people use a dilution to help cleanse and clean their crystals. It may help combat acne when used at low dilutions.

Benefits and uses

Juniper berries essential oil can help fight acne and other minor skin problems if diluted properly.

It also helps fight the cold and flu. It can help with obesity and haemorrhoids.

Main uses

- Colds
- Flu
- Acne
- Cellulite
- Gout
- Haemorrhoids
- Obesity
- Rheumatism
- Toxin Build-up

Key ingredients

- a-Pinene
- Sabinene
- B-Myrcene
- Terpinene-4-ol
- (+)-Limonene
- B-Pinene
- Gamma-Terpinene
- Delta-3-Carene
- a-Terpinene

Aromatic description

Juniper Oil is woody, sweet and fresh.

Labdanum

Cistus ladaniferus

Labdanum essential oil is also known and Cistus essential oil. It is a rich balsamic oil which is particularly used as a fixative for natural perfumes and fragrances.

It mixes well with a number of oils particularly those in the wood, spice and floral families.

Benefits and uses

Labdanum Essential Oil is used in anti-aging skin care and as an anti-inflammatory for arthritis and painful joints. It is known for its remarkable wound healing abilities.

It is great to fight against infections, especially bronchitics. It helps with coughs.

Main uses

- Antiseptic
- Anti-microbial
- Astringent
- Emmenagogue
- Expectorant
- Sedative
- Vulnerary

Key ingredients

- a-Pinene
- Camphene
- Hexen-1-ol
- Trimethylcyclohexanone
- Bornyl Acetate

Aromatic description

Labdanum Essential Oil is herbaceous, woody and with floral undertones.

Laurel Leaf

Laurus nobilis

Laurel Leaf Essential Oil is also known as Bay Laurel Essential Oil, which is not the same as bay essential oil in its properties.

It is a great oil to help with acquiring confidence and for helping with courage and focus in different tasks. It is also a great expectorant; it helps to fight colds and the flu.

Benefits and uses

Laurel Leaf Essential oil is a strong smell that can stimulate a better blood circulation. It is also used in hair care, especially to help with problems of the scalp, as dandruff.

During massages, it can also help with the relief of minor pains.

Main uses

- Amenorrhoea
- Colds
- Flu
- Loss Of Appetite
- Tonsillitis

Key ingredients

- 1,8-Cineole
- a-Pinene
- a-Terpinyl Acetate
- Linalool
- B-Pinene

Aromatic description

Laurel Leaf Essential Oil is herbaceous, fruity and fresh.

Lavender

Lavandula angustifolia

Lavender Essential Oil is one of the most popular essential oil out there. The aroma is beautiful, deep, rich and versatile. It has a deeply calming and sedative effect. It is thus a great oil to help relax, lower stress and to promote sleep.

You have to be careful when using this oil, as it has to be properly diluted to be effective and completely safe.

Benefits and uses

Lavender Essential Oil is well known for its sedative properties, but it can also greatly stimulate if it is not used properly or in too great quantities.

If used properly, it lower stress level and help with anxiety and depression. It can also be used to help with minor cuts, scrapes and little skin problems.

Main uses

- Acne
- Allergies
- Anxiety
- Asthma
- Athlete's Foot
- Cuts & Bruises
- Burns
- Chicken Pox
- Colic
- Cystitis
- Depression
- Dermatitis
- Dysmenorrhea
- Earache
- Flatulence
- Headache
- Hypertension
- Insect Bites
- Insect Repellent
- Labour Pains
- Migraine
- Oily Skin
- Rheumatism
- Scabies

Key ingredients

- Linalyl Acetate
- Linalool
- (Z)-B-Ocimene
- Lavandulyl acetate
- Terpinene-4-ol
- B-Caryophyllene
- (E)-B-Farnesene
- (E)-B-Ocimene
- 3-Octanyl Acetate

Aromatic description

Lavender Essential Oil smells floral, fresh and sweet.

Lemon

Citrus limon

Lemon Essential Oil has a very powerful and fresh lemon fragrance that really gives you energy and uplift your spirit.

When diffused, it can be really effective to clear up a bad smell in the room, such as the smell of cigarettes.

Benefits and uses

Lemon essential oil can help with colds, athlete's foot, dull skin, the flu, spots and even warts.

Main uses

- Athlete's Foot
- Chiliblains
- Colds
- Corns
- Dull Skin
- Flu
- Oily Skin
- Spots
- Varicose Veins
- Warts

Key ingredients

- (+)-Limonene
- B-Pinene
- Gamma-Terpinene
- a-Terpineol
- a-Pinene
- Geranial

Aromatic description

Lemon Essential Oil smells almost exactly like fresh lemon.

Lemon Balm

Melissa officinalis

Lemon Balm essential oil is also known as Melissa Essential Oil, which is steam distilled from the leaves and flowers of Melissa officinalis.

Lemon Balm essential oil can be helpful for acne and oily skin. It is also said to help with anxiety and support people battling with depression.

Benefits and uses

Lemon Balm essential oil can be helpful for acne and oily skin. It is also said to help with anxiety and support people battling with depression.

It generally helps with insomnia and sleep disorders as well as indigestion and nausea.

Main uses

- Insomnia
- Sleep Disorders
- Indigestion
- Nausea
- Fungal Infections
- Candida
- Viral Skin Infections
- Herpes
- Menopausal Symptoms
- Nervousness
- Stress
- Anxiety-related Symptoms
- Depression

Key ingredients

- Geranial
- Neral
- 6-methyl-5-hepten-2-one
- B-Caryophyllene
- Citronellal
- Geranyl Acetate
- Aesculetine

Aromatic description

Lemon Balm Essential Oil is very fresh, lemony and green.

Lemon Eucalyptus

Eucalyptus citriodora

Lemon Eucalyptus Essential Oil is also known as Lemon Scented Gum Essential Oil.

Lemon Eucalyptus Essential Oil has a lovely, sweet lemon aroma. It is energizing and very uplifting.

Benefits and uses

Lemon Eucalyptus Essential Oil is energizing and very uplifting. It helps with muscular injuries and skin conditions and infections.

It can also help with asthma and fevers. It also acts as an insect repellent and helps with insect bites.

Main uses

- Muscular Injury
- Fungal Skin Infection
- Bacterial Skin Infection
- Sores
- Wounds
- Respiratory Tract Conditions
- Asthma
- Fever
- Candida
- Insect Bites
- Insect Repellent

Key ingredients

- Citronellal
- Citronellol
- Isopulegol

Aromatic description

Lemon Eucalyptus Essential Oil has a lovely, sweet lemon aroma.

Lemongrass

Cymbopogon citratus

Lemongrass Essential Oil is a very sweet, fresh and lemony scent that is energizing and uplifting. It really helps give you an emotional boost and boost your productivity.

It blends extremely well with essential oils in the citrus, wood, mint and herbaceous families. However, it is very strong, so you have to be careful with the proportions.

Benefits and uses

Lemongrass essential oil gives you an emotional boost and boost your productivity.

It helps with mental, emotional and physical exhaustion and fatigue. It can also help with indigestion.

Main uses

- Muscular Aches And Pains
- Gastrointestinal Disorders
- Indigestion
- Physical And Mental Exhaustion
- Acne
- Insect Repellent

Key ingredients

- Geranial
- Neral
- Geranyl Acetate
- Geraniol
- (+)-Limonene

Aromatic description

Lemongrass Essential Oil is a very sweet, fresh and lemony scent.

Lemon Myrtle

Backhousia citriodora

Lemon Myrtle Essential Oil smells very strongly like lemons. It is a very strong anti-bacterial essential oil.

It can be used to treat acne, but it has to be very carefully diluted in order not to be dangerous when used on the skin.

Benefits and uses

Lemon Myrtle essential oil helps with indigestion, influenza and bronchitis. It is antibacterial.

Main uses

- Influenza
- Bronchitis
- Herpes Simplex
- Antibacterial
- Anti-fungal
- Sedative
- Carminative

Key ingredients

- Geranial
- Neral
- Isogeranial
- Isoneral
- 6-Methyl-5-hepten-2-one
- Linalool

Aromatic description

Lemon Myrtle essential oil has a sweet, fresh and lemony scent.

Lemon Tea Tree

Leptospermum petersonii

Lemon Tea Tree Essential Oil is anti-microbial. It has a great lemony scent and it is great for use in diffuser blends.

It can also be used in formulations for cleaning products, due to its amazing smell and its properties. It is also used in skin care, especially with acne.

It blends well with essential oils in the citrus, wood, floral, camphorous, and mint families.

Benefits and uses

Lemon Tea Tree can be used in formulations for cleaning products, due to its amazing smell and its properties.

It is also used in skin care, especially with acne.

Main uses

- Household Cleaning
- Anti-bacterial Applications
- Oily Skin
- Odors
- Insect Repellent
- Anxiety
- Stress

Key ingredients

- Geranial
- Neral
- a-Pinene
- Citronellal
- Geraniol
- Isopulegol
- Linalool
- Spathulenol

Aromatic description

Lemon Tea Tree Essential Oil has a sweet, fresh and lemony scent.

Lime

Citrus aurantifolia

Lime Essential Oil is one of the most affordable essential oils. It is very uplifting, energizing and is it great to boost your mood. It is also used to cleanse, purify and renew the spirit and the mind.

It is often used to diffuse in the house.

Benefits and uses

Lime Essential Oil is very uplifting, energizing and is it great to boost your mood.

It is also used to cleanse, purify and renew the spirit and the mind.

Main uses

- Acne
- Asthma
- Chilblains
- Colds
- Dull Skin
- Flu
- Varicose Veins

Key ingredients

- a-Pinene
- B-Pinene
- Sabinene
- Myrcene
- Limonene
- y-Terpinene
- Terpinolene
- Octanal
- Nonanal
- Tetradecanal
- Pentadecanal
- Trans-a-bergaptene
- Caryophyllene
- B-bisabolene
- Geranial
- Neryl Acetate
- Geranyl Acetate
- a-Terpineo
- Linalool

Aromatic description

Lime essential oil has a sweet, fresh and lemony scent.

Linden Blossom

Tilia vulgaris

Linden Blossom essential oil is not well known.

Caution has to be used when purchasing, to acquire it from a reliable source.

Benefits and uses

Linden Blossom Absolute can help with stress, anxiety and headaches.

Main uses

- Headache
- Insomnia
- Migraine
- Stress

Key ingredients

- Farnesol

Aromatic description

Linden Blossom Absolute is warm and floral.

Mandarin

Citrus reticulata

Mandarin Essential Oil is the sweetest and the most calming of all of the citrus essential oils.

It mixes well with many other essential oils like citrus, floral, wood, spice and herb families.

Benefits and uses

Mandarin essential oil helps to treat acne spots and skin imperfections. It can also help diminish the appearance of scars.

Main uses

- Acne
- Dull Skin
- Insomnia
- Oily Skin
- Scars
- Spots
- Stress
- Wrinkles

Key ingredients

- Limonene
- gamma-Terpinene
- a-Pinene
- B-Pinene
- B-Myrecene

Aromatic description

Mandarin Essential Oil smells sweet and citrus.

Manuka

Leptospermum scoparium

Manuka Essential Oil has many of the same properties and benefits as Australian Tea Tree Essential Oil.

However, it can be more costly. It blends well with essential oils in the wood, citrus, herbaceous, spice, mint and medicinal families. It is often a middle note in perfumes and fragrances.

Benefits and uses

Manuka essential oil helps with bronchitis, skin infections, the flu, colds, wounds and cuts.

It is also great for diffusion, perfumes and fragrances.

Main uses

- Bronchial Infections
- Bronchitis
- Catarrh
- Coughs
- Influenza
- Skin Infections
- Wounds
- Cuts
- Contusions
- Fungal Skin Infections
- Athlete'S Foot
- Parasitic Infection
- Ringworm
- Mites
- Head Lice
- Scabies

Key ingredients

- Leptospermone
- (E)-Calamenene
- a-Pinene
- Cadina-3,5-diene
- Delta-Cadinene
- a-Copaene
- Favesone
- Cadina-1,4-diene
- B-Selinene
- a-Selinene
- Isoleptospermone

Aromatic description

Manuka Essential Oil is earthy, but fresh.

Marjoram

Origanum majorana

Marjoram Essential Oil is great for aches, pain relief, minor respiratory complaints, emotional support, stress, anxiety, loss and grief.

It find blends well with a lot of other essential oils such as lavender, clary sage, rose, neroli, grapefruit.

Benefits and uses

Marjoram Essential Oil is great for aches, pain relief, minor respiratory complaints, emotional support, stress, anxiety, loss and grief.

It is used as a muscle relaxant and a sedative.

Main uses

- Muscle Relaxant
- Muscular And Abdominal Pain
- Headaches
- Menstrual And Menopausal Symptoms
- Bruises
- Gastrointestinal Disorders
- Indigestion
- Spasms
- Constipation
- Irritable Bowel Syndrome
- Diverticulosis
- Insomnia
- Stress
- Anxiety

Key ingredients

- Terpinen-4-ol
- (Z)-Sabinene Hydrate
- Linalyl Acetate
- Gamma-Terpinene
- a-Terpineol
- (E)-Sabinene Hydrate

Aromatic description

Marjoram Essential Oil has a beautiful, herbal aroma.

May Chang

Litsea Cubeba

May Chang Oil is also commonly referred to by its botanical name, Litsea Cubeba Oil.

We do not have a lot of information about this oil.

Benefits and uses

May Chang essential oil is used in fragrances and can help with digestion.

Main uses

- Acne
- Oily Skin
- Perspiration
- Indigestion

Key ingredients

- Geranial
- Neral
- (+)-Limonene
- Methyl Heptenone
- B-Myrcene
- Linalool
- Geraniol
- Sabinene
- Linalyl Acetate
- a-Pinene
- B-Pinene
- Nerol

Aromatic description

May Chang Essential Oil smells sharp.

Melissa

Melissa officinalis

Melissa Essential Oil is steam distilled from the leaves and flowers of Melissa officinalis.

Lemon Balm essential oil can be helpful for acne and oily skin. It is also said to help with anxiety and support

Benefits and uses

Melissa essential oil can be helpful for acne and oily skin. It is also said to help with anxiety and support people battling with depression.

It generally helps with insomnia and sleep disorders as well as indigestion and nausea.

Main uses

- Insomnia
- Sleep Disorders
- Indigestion
- Nausea
- Fungal Infections
- Candida
- Viral Skin Infections
- Herpes
- Menopausal Symptoms
- Nervousness
- Stress
- Anxiety-related Symptoms
- Depression

Key ingredients

- Geranial
- Neral
- 6-methyl-5-hepten-2-one
- B-Caryophyllene
- Citronellal
- Geranyl Acetate
- Aesculetine

Aromatic description

Melissa Essential Oil is very fresh, lemony and green.

Myrrh

Commiphora myrrha

Myrrh is a tree resin that has been used for centuries, especially in incense.

It is said to help with oral health. The aroma of Frankincense Oil helps to round out and freshen the aroma Myrrh Essential Oil.

Benefits and uses

Myrrh essential oil helps overall with oral hygiene and oral care. It can help the health of your gums and of your teeth.

It can also help with bronchitis.

Main uses

- Amenorrhea
- Athlete's Foot
- Bronchitis
- Chapped Skin
- Dysmenorrhea
- Gums
- Halitosis
- Hemorrhoids
- Itching
- Mouth
- Ringworm
- Toothache

Key ingredients

- Furanoeudesma-1,3-diene
- Furanodiene
- Lindestrene
- B-Elemene
- Germacrene B
- Geracrene D
- Delta-Elemene
- 2-Methoxyfuranodiene

Aromatic description

Myrrh Essential Oil smells warm, earthy and woody.

Myrrh, Sweet

Commiphora guidottii

Sweet Myrrh Essential Oil is also known as Opoponax Essential Oil which is sometimes spelled Opopanax. It is distilled from the resin from some trees.

It blends well with a lot of other oils including those in the wood, resin, spice, herbaceous, floral and citrus families.

Benefits and uses

Opoponax essential oil is antiseptic, antispasmodic, acts like an expectorant and can also be used as a fragrance fixative.

Main uses

- Antiseptic
- Antispasmodic
- Expectorant
- Fragrance Fixative

Key ingredients

- (E)-B-Ocimene
- (z)-a-Bisabolene
- a-Santalene
- (E)-B-Bergamotene
- a-Bergamotene
- Germacrene D
- Decanol

Aromatic description

Opoponax Essential Oil smells deep, resinous and woody.

Myrtle

Myrtus communis

Myrtle Essential Oil can be used for calming the mind, easing anxiety and promoting restful sleep. It is a natural sedative.

There are many types of Myrtle essential oils, but they all have the same general properties.

Benefits and uses

Myrtle Essential Oil can be used for calming the mind, easing anxiety and promoting restful sleep. It is a natural sedative. It can help with coughs, bronchitis and other respiratory issues.

Main uses

- Respiratory Issues
- Bronchitis
- Coughs
- Colds
- Fatigue
- Exhaustion
- Insomnia
- Acne
- Boils
- Hemorrhoids
- Urinary Tract Infections

Key ingredients

- a-Pinene
- 1,8-Cineole
- Myrtenyl Acetate
- (+)-Limonene
- Linalool

Aromatic description

Myrtle Essential Oil is sweet, fresh and green.

Myrtle, Lemon

Backhousia citriodora

Lemon Myrtle Essential Oil smells very strongly like lemons. It is a very strong anti-bacterial essential oil.

It can be used to treat acne, but it has to be very carefully diluted in order not to be dangerous when used on the skin.

Benefits and uses

Lemon Myrtle essential oil helps with indigestion, influenza and bronchitis. It is antibacterial.

Main uses

- Influenza
- Bronchitis
- Herpes Simplex
- Antibacterial
- Anti-fungal
- Sedative
- Carminative

Key ingredients

- Geranial
- Neral
- Isogeranial
- Isoneral
- 6-Methyl-5-hepten-2-one
- Linalool

Aromatic description

Lemon Myrtle essential oil has a sweet, fresh and lemony scent.

Nard

Nardostachys jatamansi

Nard essential oil is also known as Spikenard Essential Oil. It is great in blends, but you have to be very carefully with the proportions, as it tends to overpower then other scents in the blend.

It goes particularly well with those in the wood, spice, herbaceous and floral families.

Benefits and uses

Spikenard Essential Oil is calming and relaxing; it is sometime used to help with sleep and relaxation. It is great for meditation, prayer and other spiritual uses.

It can help with insomnia, menstrual cycle regulation and menstrual pains.

Main uses

- Insomnia
- Menstrual Problems
- Muscular Spasm
- Muscular Contractions
- Neuralgia
- Sciatica
- Bodily Congestion
- Aging Skin
- Physical Tension
- Stress-related Conditions
- Anxiety
- Nervous Tension
- Soothing
- Calming

Key ingredients

- Nardol
- Formic Acid
- a-Selinene
- Dihydro-B-ionone
- Nardol Isomer
- Selinene Isomer
- Propionic Acid
- B-Caryophyllene
- Cubebol

Aromatic description

Spikenard Essential Oil is very deep, rich, earthy and woody.

Neroli

Citrus aurantium

Neroli Essential Oil is sometimes known as Orange Blossom Essential Oil. Neroli Essential Oil is steam distilled from the wonderful blossoms of the orange tree, Citrus aurantium.

It is widely used in skin care and for its emotional benefits.

Benefits and uses

Neroli essential oil is widely used in skin care and for its emotional benefits. It helps to lower stress levels and with anxiety.

Main uses

- Depression
- Frigidity
- Insomnia
- Mature Skin
- Scars
- Shock
- Stress
- Stretch Marks

Key ingredients

- Linalool
- (+)-Limonene
- Linalyl Acetate
- (E)-B-Ocimene
- a-Terpineol
- B-Pinene
- Geranyl Acetate
- (E)-Nerolidol
- Geraniol

Aromatic description

Neroli Essential Oil is intensely floral, citrus, sweet and exotic

Niaouli

Melaleuca quinquenervia

Niaouli Essential Oil is not a scent that is appreciated by everyone. Many people think that is really does not smell good at all. It is particularly good to use it in a blend, as it reduces its particular smell.

It blends well with essential oils in the wood, mint, spice and citrus families. It is a naturally stimulating essential oil.

Benefits and uses

Niaouli essential oil is a naturally stimulating essential oil. It helps with bronchitis, coughs, throat infections and diseases and colds.

It can also help with muscular injury, acne and minor skin problems.

Main uses

- Bronchitis
- Respiratory Tract Disorders
- Influenza
- Sinus Congestion
- Sore Throats
- Catarrh
- Coughs
- Colds
- Uterine Infections
- Rheumatism
- Muscular Injury
- Rashes
- Pimples
- Acne
- Herpes
- Wounds
- Cuts
- Grazes
- Insect Repellent

Key ingredients

- 1,8-Cineole
- a-Pinene
- (+)-Limonene
- a-Terpineol
- B-Pinene
- Viridiflorol

Aromatic description

Niaouli essential oil is camphorous, earthy and a bit harsh.

Oakmoss

Evernia prunastri

Oakmoss Absolute is a base note that possesses a very deep, earthy scent.

You have to be very careful when you use it, as it can cause skin irritation when not diluted properly of use in too big quantity.

Benefits and uses

Oakmoss Absolute is almost only used in fragrances, mostly like a fixative.

Main uses

- Perfumery
- Fragrance Fixative

Key ingredients

- Methyl B-orcinolcarboxylate
- Ethyl Everninate
- Ethyl Hematonmate
- Ethyl Chlorohematommate

Aromatic description

Oakmoss Absolute is a base note that possesses a very deep, earthy aroma.

Olibanum

Boswellia carterii

Olibanum essential oil is also known as Frankincense essential oil. Frankincense is a tree resin is used for its medicinal, cosmetic, aromatic and spiritual applications.

It is used, most of the time, for spiritual uses, perfumes and incense / room fragrances. Some people seem to find the scent really grounding and calming

Benefits and uses

Frankincense Essential Oil is mostly used to mix in fragrances. It is also used in incenses, in blends or alone.

It can help get a sense of mental clarity and of general calm. It helps lower anxiety and stress levels.

Main uses

- Perfumery
- Fragrance Fixative

Key ingredients

- Methyl B-orcinolcarboxylate
- Ethyl Everninate
- Ethyl Hematonmate
- Ethyl Chlorohematommate

Aromatic description

Frankincense Essential Oil smells fresh, woody and a little spicy.

Opoponax

Commiphora guidottii

Opoponax Essential Oil is sometimes spelled Opopanax. It is distilled from the resin from some trees.

It blends well with a lot of other oils including those in the wood, resin, spice, herbaceous, floral.

Benefits and uses

Opoponax essential oil is antiseptic, antispasmodic, acts like an expectorant and can also be used as a fragrance fixative.

Main uses

- Antiseptic
- Antispasmodic
- Expectorant
- Fragrance Fixative

Key ingredients

- Methyl B-orcinolcarboxylate
- Ethyl Everninate
- Ethyl Hematonmate
- Ethyl Chlorohematommate

Aromatic description

Opoponax Essential Oil smells deep, resinous and woody.

Orange, Blood

Citrus sinensis

Blood orange Essential oil is a bit more tantalizing, bright and tart than Sweet orange Essential oil.

It has a very citrus and bright smell and the oil is derived from cold pressing its peel. It can help with a variety of issues.

Benefits and uses

Blood orange Essential oil helps with inflammation whether it is internal or external.

It has antiseptic and antibacterial properties. It is also often used to treat depression and feelings of grief. Blood orange oil can help detox the system by flushing,

Main uses

- Colds
- Constipation
- Dull Skin
- Flatulence
- Flatulence
- Flu
- Gums
- Mouth
- Slow Digestion
- Stress

Key ingredients

- Limonene

Aromatic description

Blood orange essential oil has a fruity, citrus scent.

Orange, Sweet

Citrus sinensis

Sweet Orange Essential Oil is most often called simply Orange Oil. Since it is cheap and versatile, it is one of the most popular of essential oils in aromatherapy.

If diffuse, it can help to chase away unwanted odours, such as the scent of cigarettes. Contrary to most essential oil, it is extracted by cold pressing the rinds of the orange.

Benefits and uses

Orange Essential oil helps with inflammation whether it is internal or external. It has antiseptic and antibacterial properties.

It is also often used to treat depression and feelings of grief.

Main uses

- Colds
- Constipation
- Dull Skin
- Flatulence
- Flatulence
- Flu
- Gums
- Mouth
- Slow Digestion
- Stress

Key ingredients

- (+)-Limonine
- B-Myrcene
- a-Pinene

Aromatic description

Orange essential oil has a fruity, citrus scent.

Oregano

Origanum vulgare

Oregano Essential Oil is an extremely powerful essential oil and must be used with great care.

It has to be diluted properly and used in small quantities only.

Benefits and uses

Oregano essential oil is antibacterial, anti-fungal, antiviral and an expectorant.

Is is very great to help treat the flu and colds.

Main uses

- Antibacterial
- Anti-fungal
- Antiviral
- Expectorant
- Stimulant

Key ingredients

- Carvacrol
- p-Cymene
- Gamma-Terpinene
- Thymol
- Linalool

Aromatic description

Oregano Essential Oil smells herbaceous and sharp.

Palmarosa

Cymbopogon martinii

Palmarosa Essential Oil has a slight similarity to Geranium Essential Oil. It can sometimes be used in the same way, as both the scents are very similar.

Palmarosa Essential Oil can be great to help balance dry, oily and combination skin types. You do not need to apply much to see results.

Benefits and uses

Palmarosa Essential Oil can be great to help balance dry, oily and combination skin types.

It can also be used as a spot treatment. It can help soothe anxiety and reduce stress levels.

Main uses

- Sinusitis
- Excess Mucus
- Cystitis
- Urinary Tract Infection
- Gastrointestinal Disorders
- Scarring
- Wounds
- Acne
- Pimples
- Boils
- Fungal Infection
- General Fatigue
- Muscular Aches
- Over-excercised Muscles
- Stress
- Irritability
- Restlessness
- Insect Bites And Stings

Key ingredients

- Geraniol
- Geranyl Acetate
- (E,Z)-Farnesol
- Linalool
- (E)-B-Ocimene
- B-Caryophyllene
- Geranial

Aromatic description

Palmarosa essential oil is fresh, floral and very sweet.

Palo Santo

Bursera graveolens

Palo Santo essential oil is considered very close to Frankincense Oil because both share similar constituents. It has a really overall calming and even grounding effect on most people.

It can help clear the space of any type of negative energies and replace it with good ones. This sweet scent blends well with others.

Benefits and uses

Palo Santo essential oil is used mostly for emotional and spiritual gain.

It can help calm and soothe you, and it can lower stress level and anxiety.

Main uses

- Joint Pain
- Inflammation
- General Aches And Pains
- Arthritis
- Headaches
- Allergies
- Migrain
- Stress
- Anxiety
- Panic
- Dizziness
- Nervousness
- Concentration
- Immune System Support
- Negativity
- Respiratory Infections
- Circulatory Stimulant

Key ingredients

- (+)-Limonene
- (+)-Menthofuran
- a-Terpineol
- Carvone
- Germacrene D

Aromatic description

Palo Santo Essential Oil is uniquely sweet and woody.

Parsley

Petroselinum crispum

Parsley Seed Essential Oil is mostly known for its use as a diuretic and for its ability to shrink blood vessels. Many people do not enjoy its scent, so it is best used when blended with other aromas.

You have to be careful when using it, as it can be particularly irritating.

Benefits and uses

Parsley Seed Essential Oil is mostly known for its use as a diuretic and for its ability to shrink blood vessels.

It can also help deal with indigestion and minor skin problems.

Main uses

- Depurative
- Diuretic
- Cystitis
- Uterine Tonic
- Bruises
- Amenorrhea
- Arthritis
- Cellulites
- Cystitis
- Frigidity
- Griping Pains
- Indigestion
- Rheumatism
- Toxic Build-up

Key ingredients

- Parsley Apiole
- Myristicin
- Allytetramethoxybenzene
- a-Pinene
- B-Pinene
- Elemicin
- (+)-Limonene

Aromatic description

Parsley Seed Essential Oil smells herbaceous and green.

Patchouli

Pogostemon cablin

Patchouli Essential Oil is mostly used for skin care products, but it can also be used in diffusion, mostly for emotional gains.

The smell can be quite strong and overpowering, so some people prefer to use it in blends.

Benefits and uses

Patchouli essential oil is a great asset to have in skin care. It can help with dry and oily skin, with spots, eczema and many other minor skin problems.

It can also be great in hair care and as an insect repellent.

Main uses

- Acne
- Athlete's Foot
- Chapped Skin
- Dermatitis
- Eczema
- Fatigue
- Frigidity
- Hair Care
- Insect Repellent
- Mature Skin
- Oily Skin
- Stress

Key ingredients

- Patchouli Alcohol
- a-Bulnesene
- a-Guaiene
- Seychellen
- Gamma-Patchoulene
- a-Patchoulene

Aromatic description

Patchouli Essential Oil is rich and earthy.

Pepper, Black

Piper nigrum

Black Pepper Essential oil is best used blended with other essential oils. It smells very similar to freshly ground peppercorns, but it does not have the same irritating properties and will not make you sneeze.

The best oils to mix it with would have spicy or floral notes.

Benefits and uses

Black Pepper Essential oil is used to help with circulation and can help aching muscles. It is also great to help arthritis, when properly diluted. It also helps enhance alertness and stamina to promote productivity.

It might also be useful with quitting smoking and nicotine addiction.

Main uses

- Aching Muscles
- Arthritis
- Chilblains
- Constipation
- Muscle Cramps
- Poor Circulation
- Sluggish Digestion
- Quitting Smoking and Nicotine Addiction

Key ingredients

- Limonene
- Pinene
- Myrcene
- Phellandrene
- Beta-caryophyllene
- B-bisabolene
- Sabinene
- Linalol
- Pinocarveol
- a-Terpineol
- Camphene
- a-Terpenene

Aromatic description

Peppermint Essential Oil has a very strong smell resembling peppercorns.

Pepper, Pink

Schinus molle

Pink Peppercorn Essential Oil smells a lot like freshly ground pink peppercorns, but the scent is a little more complex and rich.

It is a middle note and can help to bring together many other interesting and rich scents.

Benefits and uses

Pink pepper Essential oil is used to help with circulation and can help aching muscles. It is also great to help arthritis, when properly diluted.

It also helps enhance alertness and stamina to promote productivity. It might also be useful with quitting.

Main uses

- Arthritis
- Muscular Aches/Stiffness
- Circulation
- Sprains
- Antiseptic
- Antiviral
- Stimulant

Key ingredients

- B-Myrcene
- a-Phellandrene
- p-Cymene
- delta-Cadinene
- Limonene
- B-Phellandrene

Aromatic description

Pink Peppercorn Essential Oil has a fresh, peppery aroma.

Petitgrain

Citrus aurantium

Petitgrain Essential Oil is sometimes known as Orange Blossom Essential Oil.

Petitgrain Essential Oil is steam distilled from the wonderful blossoms of the orange tree, Citrus aurantium. It is widely used in skin care and for its emotional benefits.

Benefits and uses

Petitgrain essential oil is widely used in skin care and for its emotional benefits.

It helps to lower stress levels and with anxiety.

Main uses

- Acne
- Fatigue
- Oily Skin
- Perspiration
- Insomnia
- Stress

Key ingredients

- Linalyl acetate
- Linalol
- (+)-Limonene
- a-Terpineol
- Geranyl acetate

Aromatic description

Petitgrain Essential Oil is intensely floral, citrus, sweet and exotic.

Pimento Berry/Leaf

Pimento Officinalis or Pimento diocia

The warm, spicy aroma of Pimento Berry Essential Oil is similar to that of clove and cinnamon essential oils. The high content of Eugenol is partly responsible for this similarity. Pimento Berry Berries Pimento Berry Oil is a wonderful oil to use in the diffuser during the fall and winter.

Benefits and uses

Scientific research shows Pimento Berry has many medicinal properties. It relieves pain, eases stomach upset, and kills bacteria and fungus.

Compounds in Pimento Berry are also being investigated for use in the treatment of cancer and hypertension and is used in farming, fishing, and livestock.

Main uses

- Arthritis
- Muscle Tone
- Stiffness
- Rheumatism
- Muscular And Gastric Cramps
- Indigestion
- Nausea
- Depression
- Nervous Tension/ Exhaustion
- Neuralgia
- Coughs
- Bronchitis

Key ingredients

- Eugenol
- 1,8-Cineole
- B-Caryophyllene
- a-Caryophyllene
- Methyleugenol
- Gamma-Cadinenel
- Caryophyllene oxide

Aromatic description

Pimento Berry Essential Oil smells sharp yet is sweet with a spicy, cinnamon and clove-like aroma.

Pine, Pinyon

Pinus edulis

Pinyon Pine Essential Oil, also known as Pinion Pine Oil, and Piñon Pine Oil, is an especially fresh and aromatically pleasant pine oil.

It blends wonderfully with oils in the conifer, mint, wood and citrus families.

Benefits and uses

Pinyon Pine essential oil does not have many usages apart from the use in fragrances and perfumes.

Main uses

- Colds
- Coughing
- Flu
- Rheumatism
- Sinusitis
- Rheumatism
- Muscular Pain/Injury/Fatigue
- Gout
- Bronchial Infection
- Sinus Congestion
- General Debility
- Fatigue
- Mental And Nervous Exhaustion

Key ingredients

- Eugenol
- 1,8-Cineole
- B-Caryophyllene
- a-Caryophyllene
- Methyleugenol
- Gamma-Cadinenel
- Caryophyllene oxide

Aromatic description

Pinyon Pine essential oil is crisp and fresh.

Pine, Scotch

Pinus sylvestris

Scotch Pine Essential Oil is also known as Scots Pine Essential Oil and sometimes also Pine Essential Oil. It is produced by steam distilling the needles of Pinus sylvestris.

It is an invigorating and uplifting oil that can help fight fatigue and boost focus.

Benefits and uses

Scotch Pine Essential Oil is a good respiratory and antimicrobial oil. It is an invigorating and uplifting oil that can help fight fatigue and boost focus.

It is useful to use for colds, the flu, sinusitis, bronchitis, bronchial infection, sinus congestions and fatigue.

Main uses

- Colds
- Coughing
- Flu
- Rheumatism
- Sinusitis
- Rheumatism
- Muscular Pain/Injury/Fatigue
- Gout
- Bronchial Infection
- Sinus Congestion
- General Debility
- Fatigue
- Mental And Nervous Exhaustion

Key ingredients

- a-Pinene
- B-Pinene
- Delta-3-Carene
- B-Phellandrene
- Delta-Cadinene
- Camphene

Aromatic description

Scotch Pine Essential Oil has a crisp, fresh pine scent.

Pink Pepper

Schinus molle

Pink Peppercorn Essential Oil smells a lot like freshly ground pink peppercorns, but the scent is a little more complex and rich.

It is a middle note and can help to bring together many other interesting and rich scents.

Benefits and uses

Pink pepper Essential oil is used to help with circulation and can help aching muscles. It is also great to help arthritis, when properly diluted.

It also helps enhance alertness and stamina to promote productivity. It might also be useful with quitting

Main uses

- Arthritis
- Muscular Aches/Stiffness
- Circulation
- Sprains
- Antiseptic
- Antiviral
- Stimulant

Key ingredients

- B-Myrcene
- a-Phellandrene
- p-Cymene
- delta-Cadinene
- Limonene
- B-Phellandrene

Aromatic description

Pink Peppercorn Essential Oil has a fresh, peppery aroma.

Plai

Zingiber cassumunar

Plai Essential Oil is steam distilled from the rhizomes in the same family as ginger. It can help to manage pain, particularly for chronic conditions.

It blends really well with essential oils in the citrus, floral, mint, wood and spice families. It is an energizing oil that is especially good to use when feeling down and when you do not have any energy.

Benefits and uses

Plai essential oil It can help to manage pain, particularly for chronic conditions. It is antibacterial and can help fight various infections.

It can help with gas and flatulences, and in general with digestive issues and problems. It can also help reduce swelling.

Main uses

- Respiratory Concerns
- Colds
- Flu
- Digestive Complaints
- Gas
- Arthritis
- Joint And Muscular Pain
- Muscular Injury
- Torn Ligaments
- Muscular Spasm
- Tendonitis
- Swelling
- Menstrual Cramping
- Abdominal Spasm
- Colitis
- Diverticulosis

Key ingredients

- Terpinen-4-ol
- Sabinene
- Gamma-Terpinene
- (E)-1-(3,4-Dimethoxy-phenyl)butadiene
- a-Terpinene
- B-Pinene

Aromatic description

Plai essential oil is spicy, woody and peppery.

Ravensara

Ravensara aromatica

Ravensara essential Oil is often mixed up with Ravintsara essential Oil. Ravensara essential oil is steam distilled from the leaves of Ravensara aromatica.

We do not have a lot of accurate information about this oil.

Benefits and uses

Ravensara Essential oil can help with colds, the flu, coughs and influenza.

It can also help with joints and muscles pains.

Main uses

- Influenza
- Colds
- Bronchitis
- Other Respiratory Tract Infections
- Cold Sores
- Shingles
- Joint and Muscular Pain

Key ingredients

- Limonene
- Sabinene
- Isoledene
- Estragole
- B-Caryophyllene
- B-Myrcene
- a-Terpinene
- a-Pinene
- Linalool

Aromatic description

Ravensara Essential Oil smells slightly medicinal, eucalyptus-like.

Ravintsara

Cinnamomum camphora

Ho leaf essential oil is often times known as Ravintsara Essential Oil and it is similar to Eucalyptus oil.

It is distilled from the leaves of the same plant that gives a great variety of camphor oils.

Benefits and uses

Ho leaf essential oil can help with influenza and general helps to support the immune system.

It also helps with stress, anxiety and fatigue. It also promotes sleep.

Main uses

- Influenza
- Shingles
- Supports the Immune System
- Stress
- Depression
- Calms the Nerves
- Promotes Sleep
- Muscular Aches and Pains

Key ingredients

- 1,8-Cineole
- Sabinene
- a-Terpineol
- a-Pinene
- B-pinene
- Safrole
- Methyleugenol

Aromatic description

Ho leaf essential oil smells fresh and earthy.

Rhododendron

Rhododendron anthopogon

Anthopogon Essential oil is another name for the essential oil produced from Rhododendrons. Although not as popular as other, this essential oil compliments many other type of essential oils.

It is particularly pleasing when used with Bergamot, Clary Sage, Lavender, Rose, Virginian Cedarwood, and any essential oils comprised in the citrus, herbaceous, floral and wood families. It is a good essential oil to use to diminish stress and anxiety.

Benefits and uses

Anthopogon Essential oil is great to relieve pains from sore muscles and inflammations. It can also be used when sick to help coughs and congestion, and generally to improve the health of the lungs.

It is also useful to deal with stress and anxiety, or general emotional and spiritual in-comfort.

Main uses

- Sore Muscles
- Coughs
- Congestion
- Lungs
- Inflammation
- Emotional Discomfort
- Anxiety
- Stress
- Heart Chakra

Key ingredients

- a-Pinene
- B-Pinene
- Limonene
- Delta-Cadinene
- (3Z)-B-Ocimene
- a-Amorphene
- a-Muurolene
- p-Cymene

Aromatic description

Anthopogon Essential oil can be perceived as a floral smell with sweet undertones.

Rock Rose

Cistus ladaniferus

Cistus Essential Oil is often used as a fixative in natural perfumery and fragrance. It blends extremely well with a great quantity of other essential oils, and it brings out their scents.

It can help you feel more grounded and at peace. It is known for its great wound healing abilities.

Benefits and uses

Cistus Essential Oil is used in anti-aging skin care and as an anti-inflammatory for arthritis and painful joints. It is known for its remarkable wound healing abilities.

It is great to fight against infections, especially bronchitics. It helps with coughs issues.

Main uses

- Sore Muscles
- Coughs
- Congestion
- Lungs
- Inflammation
- Emotional Discomfort
- Anxiety
- Stress
- Heart Chakra

Key ingredients

- a-Pinene
- B-Pinene
- Limonene
- Delta-Cadinene
- (3Z)-B-Ocimene
- a-Amorphene
- a-Muurolene
- p-Cymene

Aromatic description

Cistus Essential Oil is herbaceous, woody and with floral undertones.

Roman Charmomile

Anthemis nobilis

Chamomile Essential Oil can greatly help anyone who might be struggling with depression, loneliness, intense fear, anxiety or post traumatic depression.

It is particularly effective in bringing a sense of calm and to reduce stress. It can also have a sedative effect, which helps to combat insomnia and headaches.

Benefits and uses

Chamomile Essential Oil is known to be antispasmodic, antiseptic, antibiotic and antidepressant, It can be used to bring a sense of calm and to reduce levels of stress and anxiety.

It can also have a sedative effect, which helps to combat insomnia.

Main uses

- Abscesses
- Allergies
- Arthritis
- Boils
- Colic
- Cystitis
- Dermatitis
- Dysmenorrhea
- Earache
- Flatulence
- Hair
- Headache
- Inflamed Skin
- Insect Bites
- Insomnia
- Nausea
- Neuralgia
- PMS
- Rheumatism
- Sprains
- Stress
- Wounds

Key ingredients

- Isobutyl Angelate
- Butyl Angelate
- 3-Methylpentyl Angelate
- Isobutyl Butyrate
- Isoamyl Angelate

Aromatic description

Chamomile Essential Oil is sweet, but herbaceous and fresh.

Rose

Rosa damascena

Rose Essential Oil is very helpful during times of stress and of anxiety. Rose Oil is also known to be quite helpful for insomnia and it is even considered to be an aphrodisiac. Most people really enjoy its very sweet, fresh and floral scent.

Steam Distilled Rose Essential Oil is known as Rose Otto. Solvent Extracted Rose Oil is known as Rose Absolute.

Benefits and uses

Rose Essential oil is very useful to help fight depression, anxiety and stress. It can also help with minor skin problems and menopause.

It is also used in perfumes and fragrances.

Main uses

- Depression
- Eczema
- Frigidity
- Mature Skin
- Menopause
- Stress

Key ingredients

- Citronellol
- Geranoil
- Alkenes & Alkanese
- Nerol
- Methyleugenol
- Linalool
- Citronellyl Acetate
- Ethanol
- 2-Phenylethano

Aromatic description

Rose Otto Essential Oil and Rose Absolute smell floral and sweet.

Rosemary

Rosmarinus officinalis

Rosemary Essential Oil can be used whilst cooking. It is also very useful in massage and arthritis blends. It blends really well with other oils, even though its scent is very powerful. It is a good oil for respiratory issues.

Rosemary also has a great reputation for oily skin and acne, scalp and hair care.

Benefits and uses

Rosemary essential oil helps to relieve pains, such as aching muscles and muscle cramping. It is great with skin and hair care, from oily to dry. It can help with acne and eczema.

It can also stimulate poor blood circulation.

Main uses

- Aching Muscles
- Arthritis
- Dandruff
- Dull Skin
- Exhaustion
- Gout
- Hair Care
- Muscle Cramping
- Neuralgia
- Poor Circulation
- Rheumatism

Key ingredients

- Camphor
- 1,8-Cineole
- a-Pinene
- Gamma-Terpinene
- Camphene

Aromatic description

Rosemary Essential Oil smells fresh, herbaceous, and sweet.

Rosewood

Aniba rosaeodora

Rosewood Essential Oil is also known as Bois de Rose Essential Oil. It is an extremely versatile oil that blends particularly well with woody and citrus oils.

It can also be used with more spicy and herbaceous oils. It is great when used for fragrances and perfumes, as it is sweet and floral.

Benefits and uses

Rosewood Essential Oil can help with minor skin problems, eczema and acne. It can also relieve in-comfort from insect bites, psoriasis, scarring and stings.

It can help with tonsillitis and coughs, as well as bronchitis. This polyvalent oil also helps with stress, anxiety and depression.

Main uses

- Bronchial Infection
- Tonsillitis
- Cough
- Stress Headache
- Convalescence
- Acne
- Eczema
- Psoriasis
- Scarring
- Insect Bites
- Stings
- Nervousness
- Depression
- Anxiety
- Stress

Key ingredients

- Linalool
- a-Terpineol
- (Z)-Linalool Oxide
- (E)-Linalool Oxide
- 1,8-Cineole

Aromatic description

Rosewood Essential Oil is subtle but very sweet and fruity.

Sage, Clary

Salvia sclarea

Clary Sage Essential Oil is very good for combating stress, and has a unique ability to ease stress and calm frazzled nerves. is considered an aphrodisiac by some.

It can blend very well with bergamot, lime, lavender, Roman chamomile, sandalwood, cedarwood, patchouli and rose.

Benefits and uses

Clary Sage Essential Oil is widely used in a number of topical, respiratory, digestive, emotional and feminine issues. It can help with flatulence, hair loss and dandruff.

It can also help with whooping cough and asthma attacks.

Main uses

- Acne
- Boils
- Skin Inflammation
- Hair Loss
- Dandruff
- Dry Or Mature Skin
- Muscular Aches
- Whooping Cough
- Asthma Attacks
- Eases Menstrual Pain
- Flatulence
- Intestinal Cramping
- Colic
- Stress
- Nerves
- High Blood Pressure
- Amenorrhea
- Asthma
- Dysmenorrhea
- Exhaustion
- Labor Pains
- Sore Throat

Key ingredients

- Linalyl Acetate
- Linalool
- a-Terpineol
- Germacrene D
- B-Caryophyllene

Aromatic description

Clary Sage Essential Oil is herbaceous, earthy, slightly floral.

Sandalwood

Santalum album

Sandalwood Essential Oil is a very versatile essential oil. It is particularly used in natural perfumes and fragrances, as it mixes well with other essential oils. Sandalwood is used since ancient times as incense for spiritual rituals.

It is calming and it helps to bring a general sense of well-being.

Benefits and uses

Sandalwood essential oil is great to bring calmness and a sense of inner peace to its user. It can be used against depression, to lower stress levels and to fight anxiety.

It is also great in helping with minor skin issues like acne, eczema and rashes.

Main uses

- Bronchitis
- Chapped Skin
- Depression
- Dry Skin
- Laryngitis
- Leucorrhea
- Oily Skin
- Scars
- Sensitive Skin
- Stress
- Stretch Marks

Key ingredients

- (Z)-a-Santalol
- (Z)-B-Santalol
- (Z)-Nuciferol
- epi-B-Santalol
- (Z)-a-trans-Bergamotol

Aromatic description

Sandalwood Essential Oil is rich, woody yet sweet.

Saro

Cinnamosma fragrans

Saro Essential Oil is also known as Mandravasarotra Essential Oil. It is not a very popular essential oil, but it is useful and cheaper than most oils we commonly use.

It is particularly useful for coughs, colds, headaches, respiratory complaints and to ease muscular aches and pains. It is also known to be quite stimulating

Benefits and uses

Saro essential oil is particularly useful for coughs, colds, headaches, respiratory complaints and to ease muscular aches and pains.

It can also help with digestive issues and flatulences.

Main uses

- Respiratory Support
- Soothing Allergies
- Mucus
- Congestion
- Sore Throats
- Coughs
- Bronchitis
- Coughs
- Colds
- Influenza
- Sinusitis
- Inflammation
- Natural Cleaning Blends
- Relaxation
- Catarrh
- Muscular Pain
- Muscular Injury
- Cellulite
- Wounds
- Abscesses
- Physical Exhaustion

Key ingredients

- 1,8 Cineole
- B-Pinene
- a-Pinene
- Terpinen-4-ol
- (+)-Limonene
- a-Terpineol
- Terpinyl Acetate
- Linalool

Aromatic description

Saro Essential Oil smells camphorous and a little citrus.

Tagetes

Tagetes minuta

Tagetes Essential Oil has a very fresh, sweet, floral, even fruity scent. It blends extremely well with essential oils in the citrus, floral and wood families.

Benefits and uses

Tagetes essential oil can help with corns, warts, athlete's foot, calluses, bunions and fungal infections.

Main uses

- Corns
- Warts Athlete's Foot
- Corns
- Calluses
- Bunions
- Parasitic Infestations
- Resistant Fungal Infections

Key ingredients

- (Z)-B-Ocimene
- Dihydrotagetone
- (Z)-Tagetone
- (Z)-Tagetenone
- (E)-Tagetenone

Aromatic description

Tagetes Essential Oil possesses a fresh, sweet, floral, slightly fruity aroma.

Tangerine

Citrus reticulata

Tangerine Essential Oil is fresh, sweet, citrus. It is sweeter than oranges in scent, but it has similar effects and properties.

Benefits and uses

Tangerine Essential oil helps with inflammation whether it is internal or external. It has antiseptic and antibacterial properties. It is also often used to treat depression and feelings of grief.

Tangerine oil can help detox the system by flushing unwanted toxins.

Main uses

- Stress-induced Insomnia
- Nervous Exhaustion
- Mild Muscular Spasm
- Cellulite
- Digestive Problems
- Detoxification
- Flatulence
- Constipation
- Bodily Congestion
- Fatigue
- Irritability
- Sadness
- Overly Anxious

Key ingredients

- a-Pinene
- Myrcene
- Limonene
- y-Terpinene
- Citronellal
- Linalool
- Neral
- Neryl Acetate
- Geranyl Acetate
- Geraniol
- Thymol
- Carvone

Aromatic description

Tangerine Essential Oil is fresh, sweet and citrus.

White Camphor

Cinnamomum camphora

White Camphor Essential Oil, even though it has camphor in its name, only has a very small percentage of camphor in its constituents. It is anti-inflammatory, very soothing to the skin, and it repels insects, thus preventing insect bites.

It is also useful for bruises. This very strong aroma is perfect to use in perfumes, aromatherapy and even massage oils.

Benefits and uses

White Camphor Essential Oil is anti-inflammatory, very soothing to the skin, and it repels insects, thus preventing insect bites. It is also useful for bruises. It is great for respiratory support and to help coughs and colds.

Main uses

- Muscular Aches and Pains
- Rheumatism
- Cough
- Bronchitis
- Colds
- Acne
- Rashes
- Parasitic Skin Infections
- Contusions
- Bruises
- Insect Repellent

Key ingredients

- (+)-Limonene
- p-Cymene
- a-Pinene
- 1,8-Cineole
- Sabinene
- B-Pinene
- Camphene
- Camphor

Aromatic description

White Camphor Essential Oil is a fresh but woody scent.

References

Althea Press. (2015). *Essential oils natural remedies: The complete A-Z reference of essential oils for health and healing.*

Curtis, S., Thomas, P., Johnson, F., & Neal's Yard Remedies (Firm). (2016). *Essential oils.*

Gardner, Z. E., McGuffin, M., & American Herbal Products Association. (2013). *American Herbal Products Association's botanical safety handbook.*

Lawless, J., & Roche, S. (2014). *The encyclopedia of essential oils: The complete guide to the use of aromatic oils in aromatherapy, herbalism, health & well-being.*

Lis-Balchin, M. (1999). *Aroma science: The chemistry and bioactivity of essential oils.* Guildford: Amberwood Publishing.

Sánchez, J. A. C., & Elamrani, A. (November 01, 2014). Nutrigenomics of Essential Oils and their Potential Domestic Use for Improving Health. *Natural Product Communications, 9,* 11.)

Tisserand, R., & Young, R. (2014). *Essential oil safety: A guide for health care professionals.*

Tourles, S. L. (2018). *Stephanie Tourles's essential oils: A beginner's guide.*

Worwood, V. A. (2016). *The complete book of essential oils and aromatherapy: Over 800 natural, nontoxic, and fragrant recipes to create health, beauty, and safe home and work environments.*